THE PRECONCEPTION GENDER DIET

THE PRECONCEPTION GENDER DIET

Diet A = BOY Diet B = GIRL

**Sally Langendoen, R.N.
William Proctor**

M. EVANS AND COMPANY, INC.
NEW YORK

This book is not a replacement for the medical supervision of your personal physician.

Library of Congress Cataloging in Publication Data

Langendoen, Sally.
  The preconception gender diet.

  Bibliography: p.
  Includes index.
  1. Sex—Cause and determination—Nutritional aspects.   2. Pregnancy—Nutritional aspects.
3. Menus.   I. Proctor, William.   II. Title.
QP251.L36   618.2′05   82-1470

ISBN 0-87131-372-3   AACR2

Copyright © 1982 by Sally Langendoen and William Proctor

All rights reserved. No part of this book may be reproduced or transmitted in any form or by any means without the written permission of the publisher.

M. Evans and Company, Inc.
216 East 49 Street
New York, New York 10017

Design by RFS Graphic Design, Inc.

Manufactured in the United States of America

9 8 7 6 5 4 3 2 1

Contents

Foreword	5
Introduction: The Birth of a Fascinating Idea	9
1 THE AGE-OLD QUEST TO CONTROL A BABY'S SEX	15
2 IS IT WRONG TO TRY TO CHOOSE YOUR BABY'S SEX?	26
3 SCIENTIFIC FORMULAS FOR SEX SELECTION	30
4 CAN YOU DIET YOUR WAY TO A BOY OR A GIRL?	42
5 SOME RED LIGHTS FOR WOMEN ON SPECIAL DIETS	58
6 DIET A: SIXTY-DAY DIET TO CONCEIVE A BOY	64
7 DIET B: SIXTY-DAY DIET TO CONCEIVE A GIRL	99
8 RECIPES FOR BOYS AND GIRLS	132
Conclusion: Now It's Up to You!	137
Appendix: Food Exchanges for Boy and Girl Diets	141
Bibliography	153
The Authors	157
Index	159

Foreword

THIS BOOK PRESENTS an intriguing solution to a problem that has occupied the minds of parents for generations. As a gynecologist specializing in fertility, I am especially interested in the mechanism by which such a modification in dietary intake might influence sex determination. Where would a modification of environment be most likely to act?

X- and Y-bearing spermatozoa are ejaculated in approximately equal numbers, though Dr. Landrum Shettles has pointed out that this is not necessarily always so. He has investigated the sperm population of men who have fathered large numbers of children of a single sex and believes he can see a difference in their sperm morphology consistent with the production of an excess of one or the other of the sex-determining genotypes.

The sperm are deposited in the relatively hostile acid environment of the vagina, which is made more favorable by the buffering effect of the seminal plasma and the vaginal lubricating fluids that occur as a result of sexual excitation. Sperm leave the vagina relatively quickly, having been demonstrated to be present in the much more favorable alkaline environment of the cervical mucus within thirty seconds after intercourse. Cervical mucus, which is a colloid, is a fascinating substance that demonstrates properties of both a solid and a fluid. It is a hydrophilic gel composed of a high-viscosity component, which is the gel phase, and a low-viscosity component, which consists of a variety of electrolytes and organic compounds, such as glucose, amino acids, and soluble proteins. In order to pass through cervical mucus, sperm must negotiate an obstacle course of entangled random-coiled macromolecules. They do this by the mechanical effort of their vigorously flagellating tails, which move the sperm through the meshwork and by so doing reorient the mucin macromolecules into linear channels. It is postulated that cervical mucus may provide sperm cells with energy substances required for their motility. Cervical mucus is receptive to sperm for only a short period of time during the menstrual cycle when, under the influence of high doses of estrogen, it is converted from a thick, cloudy, relatively impenetrable substance that is high in white blood cells to an abundant, clear, watery, more alkaline fluid, which is a very favorable environment for sperm.

The mechanism of sperm transport through the uterus is very little understood and is believed to involve both active and passive transport mechanisms. Substances such as prostaglandins may be involved in this process. Sperm must then cross the narrow uterotubal junctions in order to enter the fallopian tubes. This junction may act as a filtering mechanism for sperm entering the tube. Transport of sperm in the fallopian tubes to the site of fertilization is also not completely understood. How sperm manage to swim against the current created by the ciliated cells that line the fallopian tubes and all beat in the direction of the uterus is intriguing. Recently, antiperistaltic contractions of the muscle of the tube have been shown to passively transport sperm in the direction of the fertilization site.

Once sperm reach the site of fertilization, they are incapable of fertilizing the egg until they undergo a process known as capacitation. The exact nature of this process is not known, but it may involve the removal of a coating from an enzyme-active site, which is necessary for penetration of the ovum, or some other as yet unknown process. Substances in the environment of the uterus, and more especially of the tube, are necessary for this process to take place, but exactly what these substances are is unknown.

So we see that there are many hurdles sperm must overcome in order to reach the site of fertilization. Millions of sperm are deposited in the vagina. By the time the passage through cervical mucus occurs, perhaps 100,000 enter the uterus. A further marked falloff in sperm numbers occurs, so by the time the egg is reached, perhaps only from 20 to 100 sperm have survived the journey. In order for one of these sperm to fertilize the egg, the spermatozoan must penetrate the structures that surround the egg itself. These include a mass of cells that surround it in the follicle, called the cumulus, and an inner layer of these cells, called the corona radiata. The mechanism of dispersion of these cells may involve tubal factors as well as enzymes produced by the sperm themselves.

The egg is immediately surrounded by a dense translucent protein layer called the zona pellucida. The penetration of this membrane is believed to be accomplished by the release of proteolytic enzymes from the head of the sperm. Elegant microscopic preparations have shown hundreds of sperm attached to the zona with their tails beating vigorously, until one sperm succeeds in passing through the zona and rapidly attaching to the membrane of the oocyte itself. This attachment is believed to be facilitated by a substance on the membrane known as binden, which acts as a receptor for the spermatozoon. Once a spermatozoon has succeeded in attaching to the membrane, a reaction occurs and substances are released along the membrane that prevent the attachment of any other spermatozoon and, therefore, the entrance of more than one sperm into the egg. The sperm that succeeds in fertilizing the egg has now determined the sex of the conceptus.

Which of these many potential hurdles can be modified by a nutritional approach to influence sex determination in one or the other direction? Is it modification of the cervical mucus, making it more penetrable by one or the other type of sperm? Is it the tubal environment, speeding or retarding capacitation for the male- or the female-bearing sperm? Is it the penetrability of the zona, which is modified in such a way so as to facilitate its penetration by an X- or a Y-bearing sperm, but not the other? Can dietary intake really change the internal environment? The famous physiologist Claude Bernard wrote extensively about the mechanisms the body has for maintaining the constancy of the "milieu intérieur," with the kidney saving or excreting the various electrolytes so as to maintain their constant balance within the body. Are there binding sites in certain tissues where changes can be manifested at a local level? The answers to the questions raised by this book await large-scale clinical trials in which you, the reader, may participate. In addition, as our work in in-vitro fertilization progresses, we may gain additional insight into the mechanism by which a given sperm is selected for entrance into the egg. As with any method of sex selection presently available, no guarantees are given or implied. The preconception gender diet may be used by any couple who primarily desire a child, no matter what its sex may be, but who wouldn't mind trying to give the laws of chance a nudge in one direction or the other.

Charles H. Debrovner, M.D.
NEW YORK

Associate Professor of Clinical
Obstetrics and Gynecology,
New York University
School of Medicine

Lecturer, Department of Obstetrics
and Gynecology, Columbia
University College of Physicians
and Surgeons

Introduction: The Birth of a Fascinating Idea

HAVING WORKED ALL my professional life with prospective parents as a childbirth teacher and counselor, I think I've encountered almost every imaginable question and concern related to pregnancy. But the issue that provokes the most speculation and fascination is "What sex will my child be?"

Couples in my classes regularly make bets and take votes on whether a given woman will give birth to a boy or a girl. Even now, I'm recalling that just last night a young man in one of my childbirth sessions spent an inordinate amount of time examining his pregnant wife's eyeballs: He had heard something to the effect that the position of the blood vessels on the right and left sides was supposed to indicate the sex of the child his wife was carrying!

Such flights of the imagination are quite common among the majority of expectant mothers and fathers whom I've dealt with, but the interest of my students reflects something far deeper than just an idle curiosity about the unborn baby's gender. Sometimes prospective parents can get almost obsessed about which sex their baby will be because of profound emotional needs that they themselves find difficult or even impossible to put into words.

For example, many people know that they want only one or two children. And that, of course, makes each child's sex take on much more importance for them than it did for their parents or grandparents, who may have had three or more children. The fact that our national fertility rate has dropped to less than two children for each American woman indicates how widespread this trend has become.

In addition to some of the banter and flippant conversation in my classes, I hear the concern about gender being expressed in very serious personal ways among the people I counsel who are *trying* to have a child. A few years ago, my initial, unspoken response to such concern was "Why should people in this day and age be so interested in having a child of a certain sex?"

But then, as I listened more closely and thought more deeply about the subject, I realized that perhaps I was asking the wrong question. The issue wasn't really so much *why* any given person wants a boy or girl, but rather what, if anything, can be done about it? In other words, the feelings are often so profoundly rooted in a prospective parent's personality that he or she isn't interested in—or emotionally capable of—responding to any arguments for or against sex determination. All a woman may know is that she wants a girl or a boy, and she just wants you to lend a sympathetic ear to her heartfelt desires. Also, if possible, she wants some guidance about how she can *realize* those desires.

My own heart reaches out to these women, and to anxious aspiring fathers as well, because as the mother of a teenaged son, I know how intensely the entire range of maternal and paternal instincts can be felt. Sometimes it sounds silly and trivial for a man or woman to try to capture with mere words the full emotional impact of statements like: "I want a boy because I've always dreamed of playing baseball with my son," or "I want a girl because I long to be able to teach her, from my own successes and failures, how to make her way in the world," or "I want a girl because I want a chance to experience the same kind of relationship with her as my mother did with me."

But there is also another reason, besides the emotion-based ones, why this whole subject of preconception gender selection fascinates me: You see, I have a tremendous interest in good nutrition, especially nutrition for women who are thinking about getting pregnant or are already pregnant.

At first, you may think, "What on earth does good nutrition have to do with having a baby of a certain sex?" But bear with me for a moment. It's true that in the recent past, any attempt to influence the sex of a child before conception tended to focus on events that went on in the couple's bedroom, like using certain kinds of douches, assuming certain coital positions, and timing intercourse at various points during the month in relation to the woman's ovulation. Methods like these have gained a certain prominence in some segments of the medical community, and as we'll see later in this book, scientific research has validated or questioned them to one extent or another.

But there is another line of thinking that has focused on the woman's diet, rather than on her activities during intercourse. Although this research is still in the early stages of development, enough evidence is in to have convinced me that *diet does make a definite difference in the determination of a baby's sex.*

There are several reasons why the diet approach to gender selection is so exciting for me. First of all, as I've indicated, I know that having a baby of a certain sex is an important issue for many prospective parents.

Second, because I'm so concerned about good nutrition, I'm in favor of *any* diet that will raise the level of health and well-being of great numbers of aspiring mothers (many of whom seem to subsist on sodas and potato chips in their busy lives). And I've discovered that a preconception gender diet—such as the ones included in this book—may not only reward you with the sex of your choice but can also improve your health as well.

Finally, a diet approach to preconception gender selection, in contrast with some of the other methods, encourages greater spontaneity in the bedroom. Many men and women who have tried other methods of sex determination have complained that having to punctuate their passion with douching, concentrating on one coital position, or gathering all their energies for several acts of tightly scheduled intercourse can make love turn into hard labor. That kind of sex is not spontaneous. It's mechanistic!

An approach that focuses on the food you eat can free you from all this tedium. That's a large part of what excites me about this method. And since we recommend that to provide personal support the man should follow the diet as much as possible along with the woman, the diet program offers an additional possibility of increased intimacy—and also an opportunity for the prospective father to get more deeply involved in the birth process. This book, by the way, is not intended to be a substitute for professional medical advice; it is intended to suggest how through diet parents can greatly increase the possibility of determining the sex of their child. We believe that what a woman eats in the weeks immediately prior to pregnancy can play an important role in determining the sex of her baby.

While the recommended diet is safe for the vast majority of women and men, as with all diets you should see your physician prior to commencing it, explain your reason for going on the diet, and obtain medical advice. Once you find you are pregnant, your physician will recommend a pregnancy diet.

So if you're considering having a child, let me encourage you to read this book with an eye not only to learning something new about natural sex determination for your baby but also to making a personal commitment to try our approach.

And let me make one final, personal request: If you decide to participate, we'd like to hear from you *before* your baby is born, so that we can continue to contribute to the growing body of thought and research in this area. A short questionnaire and address information are provided for this purpose in the conclusion of the book.

Now let's plunge into the heart of this issue of preconception gender selection.

Sally Langendoen, R.N.

THE PRECONCEPTION GENDER DIET

The Age-Old Quest to Control a Baby's Sex

1

EVER SINCE GOD said, "Be fruitful and multiply," human beings have been preoccupied with the question of conception.

For millennia, the highest value was placed on great fertility—on having as many children as possible. As the Psalmist said, "Lo, children are an heritage of the Lord: and the fruit of the womb is his reward. As arrows are in the hand of a mighty man: so are children of the youth. Happy is the man that hath his quiver full of them." (Psalm 127:3–5, KJV)

In more recent years, as concerns like overpopulation and the high cost of rearing kids properly have come to the fore, the issue of having babies has remained a hot topic. But the questions couples ask have shifted.

Now, the most basic decision they must make is "Should we or shouldn't we?" And if they do elect to try to have children—as most husbands and wives do—they have to decide, "When should we do it, and how many should we have?"

But even as the popular childbearing notions of each age ebb and flow, one underlying issue appears to have remained constant and ever present since the very beginning: Is there any way to preselect the sex of a child?

Whether they want to have many children or only a few, couples often wish they could have some say in the number of boys or girls in their family. In one recent study conducted by Washington University in Saint Louis, 60 percent of the young married couples questioned said they would choose the sex of their children if it could be done.

There have probably been as many reasons for this desire to control a baby's sex as there have been prospective parents. Here are a few just to give you an idea:

- Husbands with a "macho" streak sometimes get obsessed with the idea of having their firstborn be a boy. And this desire may get so strong that they prefer having *all* boys, no matter how many kids come along.

- Since ancient times, a great premium has been put on having a son as an heir to the family fortune and traditions, and as the one who would carry on the family name. In the Bible, importance was placed on the birth of sons like Isaac and Jacob, who were given the responsibility of reaffirming God's covenant with His Chosen People. Thousands of years later, Henry VIII was so concerned about having a male heir that he went through a string of wives and broke with the Roman Catholic Church in his effort to sire one.

A related issue, which cropped up constantly in English common law, involved estates, which were passed on only to the male heirs of an individual. These inheritances, which were called "tail males," could not go to any female heirs. So if a couple gave birth only to girls, the future of all their material possessions could be placed in jeopardy. As you might imagine, when a husband and wife in this situation neared the end of childbearing age, they were tempted to try every farfetched selection method they could find to conceive a boy—and save their estate.

■ Women, as well as men, have a strong desire for a male firstborn, according to recent research. In one analysis of the 1970 National Fertility Study conducted by the Office of Population Research at Princeton University, it was determined that 63 percent of women without children want a boy baby first.

■ Both men and women may want a boy *or* a girl, or a certain proportion of boys and girls, because their own families were that way—or they *wish* they had been that way!

■ Some couples are indifferent about the sex of their *first* child. But if they plan on limiting their family to only two kids, they may develop a strong desire for a child of the opposite sex the second time around, just to "balance things out."

In a study of the attitudes of young married couples toward predetermination of their children's sex, Saul Rosenzweig and Stuart Adelman of Washington University in Saint Louis found that 91 percent of those desiring two children wanted one boy and one girl. Also, of the entire group studied—some of whom wanted more than two children—69 percent wanted an equal number of boys and girls.

■ Some women, on the other hand, have an overwhelmingly strong desire for a female firstborn. For example, in a number of cases the mother may sense a need to have a daughter who, it is hoped, will be a companion and confidante for the rest of the mother's life. Or sometimes the desire for a girl stems from feminist considerations—such as an urge to create a supersuccessful female prototype who is free of the mother's emotional weaknesses.

■ From a more scientific perspective, some modern women are aware that they are carriers of sex-linked disorders that may be passed on to any males they conceive. For example, there are forms of hemophilia, diabetes, muscular dystrophy, and certain enzyme-deficiency conditions that a mother may pass on to a son—but not to a daughter. In such cases, the woman may well want to give birth to girls only.

This list of reasons why people might want to select the sex of their children could go on for many more pages. But by now the key point should have become obvious: A significant number of people want to choose their baby's gender. Now, the question becomes: Is there any way to go about it?

A massive body of folklore has grown up over the ages that purports to inform parents how they can conceive a boy or girl. Some of the notions are obviously pure fantasy, with no basis at all in reality. Others, as we'll see, may have some element of validity.

But before we get into any evaluations, let's take a look at some of the sex-selection techniques that have popped up in the prescientific past:

- In Ghana, on the west coast of Africa, eating boiled oysters, without the salt water solution in which they were prepared, is supposed to predispose a mother to have a girl. Eating salted fish, on the other hand, is supposed to enhance the mother's chances of conceiving a boy.
- Hippocrates, the "father of modern medicine," advised that tying off the prospective daddy's right testicle before intercourse would result in the birth of a boy. Conversely, tying off the left testicle would result in the birth of a girl.
- Other early Greeks are reported to have believed just the opposite—that tying off the left testicle would produce a boy, because male sperm came predominantly from the right side.
- Expanding rather rashly upon these teachings, some eighteenth-century French noblemen subscribed to the practice of *cutting off* the left testicle to enhance their chances of siring a boy.

- The mandrake root, a stemless perennial herb that often grows in uncultivated fields in the eastern Mediterranean, is shaped somewhat like a man and has been regarded, through the ages, as an aphrodisiac and a source of fertility—especially fertility that would lead to the birth of a male child. For example, in Genesis 30:14–20, the childless Rachel was desperate to give her husband, the Hebrew patriarch Jacob, a child, and especially a son. So she traded to her rival, Leah, Jacob's other wife, her opportunity to have intercourse with Jacob in return for some mandrakes.
- Like the mandrake, the ginseng root, a perennial herb which grows in North America and the Far East, vaguely resembles a man, with arms, legs, and a male sexual organ. Sometimes called "the man root," this plant was considered by American Indians and others to be a powerful source of fertility if consumed by a woman who wanted to bear a boy.
- Eating two fruits that have grown together will increase the probability that a woman will bear twins. An interesting twist on this legend in some South American countries is that the prospective father who eats two bananas that have merged will cause his wife to bear twins.
- Male Latin lovers are more potent than men from the "cooler" countries and have a better chance of impregnating a woman with a boy.
- The more hair a man has on his body, the more likely he will be to cause his sexual partner to have a strapping son.
- Wearing certain colors during pregnancy will help determine the baby's sex. The most popular tradition in this regard, which has permeated the Western countries, is that wearing pink will result in a girl, while blue will lead to a boy.
- In Czechoslovakia and Hungary, there is a tradition that if a woman wants a son, she should place poppy seeds on her windowsill; if she wants a girl, sugar should be used instead of the seeds.

- In ancient Rome, lettuce was thought to be a powerful source of sexual desire and fertility for women who wanted sons. If you could take a time machine back to an old Roman wedding banquet, you'd find more lettuce on the table than you might have a taste for!
- In some sections of the rural United States, childless women were told they could greatly increase their chances of bearing children in general, and boys in particular, if they would throw some cowpeas across a local street—and also include substantial portions in their daily menus.
- There's a superstition in England that if a daughter is born while the moon is fading from sight, the next child will be a son. On the other hand, a son who arrives with the fading moon will portend a girl the next time around.
- In the fifth century B.C., the Greek Parmenides advised aspiring mothers to lie on their right sides during coitus because male babies were conceived on the right side. As with the testicle theories, however, there is a difference of opinion here. Other "experts" have advocated having intercourse on the left side for a boy.
- During the Middle Ages, certain church officials would prescribe a drink of lion's blood and wine for a woman and then direct her to have intercourse under a full moon if she wanted to have a son.
- According to Aristotle, the sex of the child depended on which partner was sexually the most potent and vigorous. Also, he believed that climatic conditions had an impact: "More males are born if copulation takes place when a north wind rather than a south wind blows, for the south wind is moister."
- Certain magical chants recited before intercourse are thought in some cultures to help produce male babies.
- Wearing boots to bed has at times been a popular male-child method in parts of Europe.
- Coitus during the rising of the tide (like the waning of the moon) will result in a boy.

- There is one school of thought, including a scientist or two, that says drinking a bicarbonate of soda will result in a son.
- According to another tradition, popular in some parts of the United States, babies conceived in warm weather will probably be girls and those conceived in cold weather are more likely to be boys. (Don't laugh: One Illinois physician has investigated birth ratios under different weather conditions in Chicago and Detroit and has come to substantially this very conclusion.)
- The sexual partner who is the more relaxed tends to produce an offspring of his or her own sex. There has been some research recently that tends to support this conclusion. Donald and Locky Schuster of Iowa State University have studied a limited sampling of women raped by men and their offspring and have found that 90 percent of the children conceived out of rape were boys. Their conclusion: The parent who is under the lesser amount of stress (in rape, this was assumed to be the man) tends to produce a child of his or her own sex.
- In other cultures, from the South Sea islands to the mountains of Europe, strange formulas have at various times prevailed—such as a young woman sleeping with a little boy just before her wedding, a wife dressing in man's clothes before coitus, and a husband taking an ax to bed with him during intercourse.
- Diet-oriented theories have also appeared regularly in different cultures: In sections of central and southern Europe, it's believed that a successful nut harvest signals the birth of more male children. In many parts of the world, a woman is encouraged to eat salty steaks, roasts, fish, and other meats high in protein if she wants a boy; also, any sharp or sour foods will enhance her chances for a son. Other favorite "male-child" foods have included the sex organs of different animals, leafy vegetables prepared with olive oil and salt solutions, and low-carbohydrate items. For a daughter, on the other hand, a diet high in sweets and carbohydrates has at various times been recommended.

■ One of the most interesting and complex of the traditional sex-selection techniques comes from an ancient Hebrew tradition. This approach is based on various talmudic interpretations of a clause in Leviticus 12:2, which reads, "When a woman gives birth and bears a male child . . ." (New American Standard Bible). One English translation of the Hebrew Masoretic text renders the phrase *gives birth* as "be delivered," and other translations make it "conceives."

But there is also one line of rabbinic thought that prefers to translate that phrase as "emits semen" or "emits seed," and this is the source of the sex-selection theories.

In the Babylonian Talmud, one Rabbi Isaac, referring to a Rabbi Ammi, said that the clause in Leviticus 12:2 really means that if a woman emits semen first, she will bear a male child. On the other hand, if the man emits his semen first, the offspring will be a girl.

Rabbi Isaac cites 1 Chronicles 8:40 to the effect that Ulam's sons were mighty warriors and archers, and had many sons, and grandsons. Then he asks, "Now is it within the power of man to increase the number of sons and sons' sons?"—in effect, the same question we're exploring in this book, except we would also say, "daughters and daughters' daughters?"

The rabbi's answer is that they could preselect their male offspring "because they contained themselves during intercourse, in order that their wives should emit their semen first."

To understand and evaluate this technique, however, it's necessary to ask next, what exactly did it mean to these ancient rabbis for the woman to "emit semen"?

Dr. Fred Rosner, in the *Israel Journal of Medical Sciences*, believes that the phrase could have referred either to the woman's ovulation or to a female orgasm, and he concludes it must have been the latter. Otherwise, he says, it wouldn't have made any sense to talk about the man restraining himself during intercourse in order to allow the wife to "emit semen" or "emit seed" first.

Rosner argues that the best interpretation of the concept of a woman's "emitting semen" would be that she had orgasm *before* her husband and thereby produced male offspring. He goes on to conclude that this interpretation agrees with certain modern medical research. More specifically, he says, it's known that orgasm increases the flow of alkaline secretions in the woman, and this alkaline bodily environment is considered by some researchers to be a more favorable environment for male sperm. Hence, if the woman has her orgasm first, she may be more likely to have a boy.

This list of ancient sex-selection techniques, some supported in part by scientific research and some having no connection whatsoever with science, could go on indefinitely. But we've looked at enough of them to see that the human imagination has been working overtime through the ages to come up with a reasonably reliable way to preselect a boy or a girl baby.

The main issue—trying to control the gender of the child—has also spawned a number of secondary concerns. One of these has been a search for techniques merely to learn in advance or predict what the sex of the baby will be.

The most common and scientifically reliable method today is amniocentesis, or the insertion of a needle into the pregnant womb to extract amniotic fluid from which to grow a culture. But this approach is only the last and most reputable in a long line of folk-medicine techniques.

For example, if the mother is carrying her baby high in the womb, that's supposed to indicate she'll have a boy. If the fetus is low, it's a girl. According to one Welsh superstition, you can tell the sex of a baby before birth by hanging a shoulder of mutton over the back door to the couple's home. If a man enters the door first, the child will be male; and if a woman comes in, it will be female.

But perhaps one of the most popular folk methods of relatively recent vintage in the United States is the so-called "Drano test." The idea here is to put a half-inch or so of Drano at the bottom of a glass or cup, and then have the pregnant woman spit into it. (One variation on this approach is to add Drano to the woman's urine.) If the Drano crystals turn brown, she'll have a boy; if they stay clear, she'll give birth to a girl.

At least one doctor in New York—who shall go unnamed—swears (privately) by this test, and he claims the results have been 100 percent accurate with his patients. But he's in a distinct minority in the medical profession, where this technique is generally regarded as rank superstition. Also, there are possible dangers with the test, because Drano, which has a powerful and sometimes almost explosive action in clearing clogged-up drains, can burn or otherwise injure the unwary user.

One woman who tried the Drano test in New York made the mistake of spitting too hard into her cup, with the frightening result that some of the Drano dust blew up into her eyes. She immediately washed her eyes and face in a long shower, and there was no injury, but the result might easily have been much more tragic.

The dangers were also pointed up in one of Ann Landers's popular newspaper advice columns entitled " 'Drano test:' Down the Drain." Miss Landers ran several letters speaking out against the test, including one from the Drano company itself. In one case, a woman had added Drano to her urine, which she had put into a glass container. But the glass "exploded in a zillion pieces."

Despite what that one New York doctor says about the reliability of the test, there's no scientific support for it. And the dangers accompanying this method seem to far outweigh the remote possibility that you may learn a few months in advance what sex your baby will be.

Even amniocentesis has some dangers. There have been cases where the fetus has been inadvertently injured by a misdirected needle. And even the widely hailed scientific reliability of amniocentesis has been known to fall sadly short.

For example, in an article in *The New York Times* entitled

"It's Not Nice to Be Fooled by Mother Nature," the author, Joan Gage, details how her doctor tested her by amniocentesis and assured her she would have a boy. But then when she woke up from the anesthetic after her Caesarean delivery, the doctor said, "Congratulations! You have a healthy baby *girl*."

Despite Gage's experience, amniocentesis is, generally speaking, quite reliable as a *predictor* of a child's sex. Unfortunately, the same can't be said for the various folk and traditional techniques we've examined that focus on the more important issue—*selecting* the baby's gender.

But there *has* been a definite increase in the reliability of certain methods that claim to enhance your chances of having a boy or girl. And in just a moment we'll plunge into the nuts and bolts of how those methods work and what your chances of success with them may be.

But first, it's important to be absolutely sure that you really *want* to pick your child's sex. To resolve this issue, let's now consider briefly some of the moral and ethical implications of preconception sex selection.

2 Is It Wrong to Try to Choose Your Baby's Sex?

SUPPOSE THAT YOU'VE happened upon a reasonably reliable way to choose your baby's gender before it's born. Then, imagine someone asks you, "Are there any moral or ethical problems with this idea of selecting your baby's sex?"

Your first thought may be "Of course not—you just decide whether you want a girl or a boy, and you do it!" But the issue is not quite as simple as that. A blanket approval of *all* sex-selection techniques can get you into a moral morass that you may have some difficulty escaping from.

For example, up to this point we've been talking about *pre*-conception selection of your baby's gender. But there are also *post*conception ways to go about this gender determination, and it's extremely important to distinguish between the two because the moral problems involved in each are vastly different.

Actually, the only method of postconception sex selection is abortion.

As it stands now, most obstetricians have a negative reaction to terminating a pregnancy if the request is made just because the pregnant woman has decided she doesn't want a child of a particular sex. One of the reasons for this reluctance is that the amniocentesis technique cannot reveal the sex of the fetus with acceptable accuracy until the woman is about eighteen weeks into her pregnancy. And abortions performed this late in pregnancy can be unsettling.

One way of getting around this problem of postconception sex selection through *late* abortion may be a method that has been reported by the Chinese, who are developing a procedure for much *earlier* fetal sex identification. By inserting a device into the woman's cervix and taking out some cells, the Chinese doctors have been able to correctly detect the sex of the fetus 94 percent of the time—and to do it within two months of conception.

But there are still plenty of problems with this method, even though it's easier on the mother-to-be. For one thing, spontaneous miscarriages occurred in 4 percent of the cases. And there's something else that's disturbing from an ethical point of view: Of the thirty pregnancies that were voluntarily terminated, twenty-nine involved female fetuses.

In contrast to the postconception approach, selecting a child's sex *before* conception presents fewer problems. Some religious groups may worry about some of the preconception techniques, like sperm separation or artificial insemination, "toying too much with nature." But many of the other preconception methods—like timing intercourse to coincide with a certain part of the woman's ovulation cycle, favoring certain coital positions, and adjusting the diet—are so "natural" that they shouldn't present any problems to major religious traditions.

This is not to say that the idea of picking a baby's sex is completely unobjectionable to everybody—just that there seem to be fewer people who would actively oppose the idea. Feminists will probably still rise up in arms at the first suggestion of a significant popular movement to preselect a baby's gender. And a number of social scientists would join them in their opposition.

One basis for this opposition would be the fact that some polls show a preference among both women and men for male babies over females, especially when the couple is childless. As a result, if it were possible to preselect the sex of a child reliably now, the impact over the short term, say the next few years, could well be a 20 percent increase in male births, according to a study conducted by Charles Westoff of Princeton and Ronald Rindfuss of the University of Wisconsin.

Westoff and Rindfuss believe this sexual imbalance in the population would level out after a few years, so the ratio of male to female births by preconception sex-selection techniques would be virtually identical to what it is now with uncontrolled, random births. (Currently, there are about 105 boys born for every 100 girls.)

But such assurances would not convince feminists or even some social scientists, some of whom argue that preconception selection in favor of males might help solve the world population problem because there would be fewer women around to bear children.

Feminist writer Eva Figes speculates in *Ms.* magazine: "A largely male population would lead to forms of social unrest which would be all too explicable. We would need another Vietnam War to take care of all the restless, rootless males, or some other modern crusade of equally major proportions. How about a crusade to bring the true pill to the heathen lands of the unconverted? The flag could bear a large red Y on a white ground, instead of the old true cross." (The Y, by the way, refers to the Y-bearing sperm that produce boy babies—but more about that later.)

Social scientists, however, tend to worry about social disruptions of a type somewhat different from what Eva Figes describes. For example, some concern has been expressed that too many males in the population might lead to increased male homosexuality and perhaps even polyandry (a marriage form in which one woman has two or more husbands at the same time).

Also, since many studies show a strong preference for having a male child first, a reliable sex-selection method might have a decisive impact on political and social leadership and the future content of sex stereotypes: Firstborn children—male or female—tend to be higher achievers and more success-oriented than their younger siblings. And some studies have even shown that they have, on average, higher IQs than the younger kids. Hence, women who are still struggling for equal treatment in many areas of the working world might be irremedially handicapped if few of them have the advantage of being the first child in a family.

In addition, there are medical objections to the movement to develop ways to choose a baby's sex—particularly if the choices tend to favor sons over daughters. For one thing, males seem to have a less hardy physical makeup than females: On the average, they contract more serious, life-threatening diseases and die earlier. With many more males in the population as a result of sex selection, the whole human population might be weakened.

Also, there is a prevailing belief that boys and men tend to be more combative than girls and women. If this is true, and the number of males in the population increases significantly, we might find ourselves confronting a much higher crime rate and the threat of more wars around the world.

As you can see from this brief survey of some of the moral and ethical implications of being able to select a child's sex, the issue isn't as clear-cut as it might seem at first blush.

Some of our readers may have already decided, after this discussion of the ethics of the issue, that they're not interested in pursuing the subject any further. But many others probably want to continue the investigation, perhaps with the idea of eventually trying to influence the gender of their own future children.

So now let's take a look at some of the major scientific advances in preconception sex selection and see which ones you might be able to use right now in your own family planning.

Scientific Formulas for Sex Selection 3

A GREAT DEAL has been written by scientific researchers on possible ways to increase your chances of having a boy or a girl. And preliminary results suggest that some of the methods tested *do* work, at least up to a point.

Before we get into the details of some of these scientifically tested techniques, it's necessary first to recall the basics of how conception takes place. A baby's sex is completely dependent on which of the two types of sperm penetrate the woman's egg after sexual intercourse.

The reason for this is that the woman's egg has only X chromosomes, which are female chromosomes. The man's semen, on the other hand, contains two types of sperm: those having only X (female) chromosomes (called X or female sperm), and those having *both* X and Y (male) chromosomes (called Y or male sperm). So if an X sperm penetrates (or fertilizes) the woman's egg, the child will be a girl; and if a Y sperm gets to the egg first, the child will be a boy.

The X (female) sperm are larger, heavier, and slower than the Y (male) sperm, and they operate best in an acidic environment. The Y sperm, on the other hand, are smaller and quite mobile and get along better in an alkaline environment. These differing characteristics of the X and the Y sperm, as we'll see, become quite important in some of the preconception sex-selection techniques.

The sperm can retain their power to fertilize an egg for two to four days after they've been deposited inside the female during intercourse. On the other hand, the woman's egg can exist only for up to one full day after ovulation. If conception takes place, it usually occurs after the sperm swim up through the woman's cervix and uterus and meet the egg in the ducts (oviducts or fallopian tubes) just off the uterus.

Now that you've had this little "refresher course" in how conception takes place, let's look at a few of the methods that modern science has tested to influence whether an X or a Y sperm has the best shot at the woman's egg. Each of these techniques has its backers *and* its critics. But the chances are that several—or all— of them have some degree of validity. So they're worth considering seriously and in some detail if choosing the sex of your next baby is at all important to you.

1. **THE DOUCHE METHOD.** A German medical scientist named Felix Unterberger decided to take information gained through veterinary research and apply it to his human patients who were infertile. He had them use a 2 percent sodium bicarbonate solution in a douche just before intercourse. The result: They gave birth—to male infants.

He decided there must have been something in that douche that not only overcame the infertility but also produced so many boys. So he staged a full-fledged test for those women who specifically wanted boys, and fifty-three out of the fifty-four in his test who conceived did, indeed, have male infants. He also tried to get a second group to use a lactic acid and vinegar douche, or a lemon juice douche, in an effort to produce daughters. But according to Dr. A. D. G. Gordon in *Nursing Times*, he couldn't get enough takers to conduct the test.

Other researchers tried similar techniques. Then, Dr. Landrum B. Shettles of Columbia University came along and made the douche one of the key elements in a sex-selection procedure. He popularized this whole "package" more than a decade ago.

He believed that women who wanted boys should use an alkaline douche, consisting of two tablespoons of baking soda in a quart of water, just before intercourse. Those who wanted a girl should use an acidic douche, made up of two tablespoons of white vinegar in a quart of water, just before intercourse.

The purpose of the douche was to change the pH, or acid-alkaline balance, in the woman's vagina so that either male sperm (in an alkaline environment) or female sperm (in an acidic environment) would be favored.

But the douche method has come under heavy fire by other scientists. Several experiments have been conducted with both human and animal sperm, and the scientists performing those tests have concluded that the pH in the vagina has no impact on the viability of the X or Y sperm—and hence no influence on whether a woman conceives a girl or a boy.

Still, despite the disagreements, there are those, like Elizabeth Whelan, a sex-selection advocate and the author of *Boy or Girl?*, who feel that there is some chance the douche method may have an impact on the sex of the baby and that, all things considered, it probably "doesn't hurt to try."

2. ORCHESTRATING THE ACT OF INTERCOURSE.
Reputable medical people have also recommended that

couples interested in conceiving a child of a particular sex should pay attention to the way that they go about having intercourse.

For example, there are many experts who favor trying the old talmudic method recommended by the rabbis we discussed in the first chapter. With that approach, if a boy is desired, the woman should reach orgasm before the man. In this way, some argue, the vaginal and reproductive organs are more likely to be permeated with alkaline substances that are more hospitable to the male sperm. Conversely, if the woman doesn't have an orgasm, her vagina is more likely to be more acidic—and girls may result.

Another intercourse-related technique involves the use of certain coital positions. Dr. Landrum Shettles and his collaborator, David Rorvik, argue in their book *Your Baby's Sex: Now You Can Choose* that to conceive a girl, the couple will have the best chance with the face-to-face, or "missionary," position of intercourse. With this method, Dr. Shettles says, the sperm will have a better chance of being released *away from* the opening of the cervix (the entrance to the womb) and more into the acid secretions of the vagina.

For a boy, on the other hand, Shettles believes it's best for the man to penetrate the woman from the rear so that the sperm will be deposited right at the cervix. The secretions in this part of a woman's body are more likely to be alkaline, and hence more favorable to the Y (male) sperm.

There are several corollaries to this coital-position approach, according to Shettles and other medical researchers who have tested his technique: First of all, it's important for the man to achieve a deep penetration at the moment of male orgasm if the couple wants a boy, and shallow penetration if they want a girl. Deep penetration gets the sperm closer to the alkaline cervix, while shallow penetration puts them into the more acidic sections of the vagina.

Also, the husband should abstain from intercourse for at

least a week before the attempt is made to conceive. This abstention is supposed to increase the total amount of sperm in his body and thus give the large number of fast Y (male) sperm an advantage in their race to reach the woman's egg. In support of this theory, some studies have indicated that frequent intercourse, which keeps the male sperm down, tends to favor the conception of females.

3. **THE TIMING OF INTERCOURSE.** This method of preconception sex selection is one of the most popular—and most controversial—being bruited about these days.

In the first place, there are two distinct schools of thought among those who believe that scheduling the sex act for certain times of the month is a valid approach to gender control. The first group, represented most prominently during the past decade by Shettles, believes that if you want a boy, you should try to have intercourse at the time of the woman's ovulation. For a girl, according to the Shettles school, intercourse should cease two to three days before ovulation.

The point of ovulation can be estimated in several ways. One approach is to keep track of the number of days that have passed since the beginning of the woman's previous menstrual period (usually ovulation occurs about fourteen or fifteen days before the beginning of her next period).

Another way to estimate when ovulation is about to occur is for the woman to keep meticulous track, over several consecutive months, of shifts in her body temperature with a sensitive basal thermometer (you can buy one in your local drugstore for a modest sum). Ovulation usually takes place a couple of days before the biggest rise in her temperature during the month.

Shettles has reported 80 percent success in clinical testing of his *complete* procedure for preconception sex determination. His entire package, of which timing of intercourse is the centerpiece, can be summarized this way:

To conceive a boy:
1. Time coitus at the moment of ovulation.
2. Use an alkaline douche before intercourse.
3. The woman should experience orgasm before the man.
4. Vaginal penetration should be from the rear.
5. The man should penetrate the woman deeply as he ejaculates.
6. The man should abstain from intercourse for several days before the conception try.

To conceive a girl:
1. Time coitus two to three days before ovulation.
2. Use a vinegar douche.
3. The woman should avoid orgasm.
4. The couple should use the face-to-face coital position.
5. The man should penetrate shallowly during intercourse.
6. The man should have frequent ejaculation just prior to the conception attempt.

Shettles at one point became so certain of the validity of his approach that he even went so far as to say, "I believe that if the couple is conscientious with the douche and the timing that they can achieve success 85 to 90 percent of the time."

The Shettles technique has found a number of supporters, some of whom report having conducted medical tests and studies that uphold his results. For example, Dr. Cedric S. Vear reported in late 1977 in the *Medical Journal of Australia* that he had succeeded ten consecutive times in achieving the desired infant sex by using the Shettles approach. He noted that the chances of attaining this success rate in ordinary, random intercourse would have been 1 in 1,024—or practically impossible.

But the Shettles school also has many detractors. One outspoken opponent is Elizabeth Whelan, who has written a number of books and articles on sex education, population, and nutrition. Relying on research done by Dr. Rodrigo Guerrero of the University of Valle in Colombia, South America, she has concluded that the timing of intercourse is an essential factor in trying to control the sex of the child. But she believes that the Shettles approach to timing is 180-degrees wrong.

Or, as she puts it in her book *A Baby? . . . Maybe*, Shettles's recipe "was based on the experience of women who were artificially inseminated. It is known that women who are artificially inseminated prior to ovulation are more likely to have girls, and those inseminated at ovulation are more likely to have boys. *We now know that just the opposite is true when babies are conceived the natural way.*"

According to Guerrero, if you want to have a boy, you should have intercourse four or more days before ovulation. If you want a girl, time your crucial coitus for one day before ovulation. Whelan claims that the Guerrero method will increase your odds from 50 percent to 68 percent for having a boy baby, and from 50 percent to 56 or 57 percent for having a girl.

But not everybody has rushed to agree that Guerrero has found the key. For their part, Shettles and his collaborator, David Rorvik, responded in a later book, *Choose Your Baby's Sex*, that their entire sex-control package—with the douching, coital positions, and so on—*simulates* artificial insemination, and thus is still valid.

Other medical researchers have suggested that *both* the Shettles and the Guerrero theories may have some holes in them. In one attempt to employ the Shettles concept in an experiment in Singapore, Nancy Williamson, T. H. Lean, and D. Vengadasalam issued nearly 11,000 invitations to join a sex-preselection clinic. But less than one-tenth of those invited attended the clinic more than once. Of those who came back more often, the large majority resisted complying with the entire Shettles "package" of timing intercourse, douching, and the other suggested techniques.

Only forty-five of the women in the Singapore experiment actually became pregnant. Thirty-one births had occurred by the time the test was recorded in a medical journal, and *all* those new mothers had wanted boys. But only fourteen of the infants, or fewer than the number expected from the usual boy-girl ratio in the general population, *were* boys.

As the researchers pointed out in their report, the results they came up with don't support the position of either Shettles or Guerrero. Only six of the women who gave birth reported using Shettles's method completely correctly. Of those, four (or two-thirds) obtained a child of the sex they wanted (a boy) and two didn't. But these numbers are too small to serve as the basis for any generalizations.

In the remaining cases, the women followed only part of the Shettles program, such as using the douche but failing to time the moment of intercourse correctly.

Their reasons for not following the required procedures are perhaps the most significant point of all because they show how difficult it is to give the complex Shettles program a "good run for its money."

As Williamson and her colleagues report in the *Journal of Biosocial Sciences*, "Almost all respondents mentioned they had problems in taking and recording their temperatures daily. Next in difficulty was the douching. Half of the women mentioned having difficulty douching before having intercourse. . . . About a quarter of the women were not sure when ovulation was supposed to occur in relation to the temperature shift. Almost half of the women mentioned lack of cooperation from their husbands as a problem. The most common reason for stopping use of the method was pregnancy; the next most common was lack of interest (or faith) in the method."

In other words, even if the Shettles method improves

your chances to have a boy or girl, it imposes too many rules and restrictions on the fundamentally passionate act of intercourse. So it may be that the average couple is unlikely to follow the program to the letter—and especially not if it takes more than a month or two to achieve pregnancy.

And finally, as we've already seen, Guerrero disagrees with Shettles on the best time to have intercourse to increase your chances of having a boy or girl. But then, there are those who disagree with Guerrero.

For instance, Dr. Robert Glass, of the department of obstetrics and gynecology at the University of California School of Medicine in San Francisco, says that the way Guerrero timed ovulation varied from one experiment to the next. As a result, Glass says, it's not apparent exactly when the temperature rise, which signals ovulation, actually occurred in the tests.

If all this sounds confusing, rest assured that many of the medical experts are as confused as you are. The test results are conflicting and inconsistent, and the best that can probably be said about any of these techniques is that it *may* increase the odds you'll have a boy or a girl. But at this point, it seems equally clear that none of the procedures discussed thus far can be classified as highly reliable.

Also, the difficulty of adhering strictly even to the requirement of trying to time the woman's ovulation—much less going along completely with Shettles's douching/coital-position program—will just be too much for many couples to take.

Having a baby of a certain sex may be fairly important to many husbands and wives. But having a relaxed, enjoyable sex life is a much higher priority.

4. **SEPARATING THE MALE AND FEMALE SPERM IN ARTIFICIAL INSEMINATION.** This method of preconception gender selection is perhaps potentially the most reli-

able and promising—at least from a purely scientific point of view.

Right now, the research in this area is still in a preliminary stage, but there are several indications that medical researchers are having some degree of success with humans. In 1973, Ronald J. Ericsson, then a scientist with a Berlin company who subsequently moved to California, formulated a method to separate the Y (male) sperm from the X (female) sperm outside the body.

To put it in the simplest terms, he collected a semen sample and injected the sperm into a solution that was difficult for the sperm to swim through. The fastest sperm (the Y, male sperm) swam to the bottom of the solution first, and their accumulation resulted in a Y-rich sperm sample.

Another scientist, W. Paul Dmowski, director of the fertility unit at Michael Reese Hospital and Medical Center in Chicago, then took the process one step further. After studying Ericsson's work, he concluded quite logically that the Y-rich sperm should produce more boys than girls. So he conducted an experiment with women who wanted boy babies.

First of all, he found forty-five women who were interested in participating in the test and collected samples of their husbands' sperm. Then, using a variation on Ericsson's method, he separated out a high proportion of the Y sperm from the samples so that he got a new semen concentration of about 84 percent Y sperm. Finally, he introduced this concentrated male semen into the wives—with the result that about 75 to 80 percent of those who conceived gave birth to boys.

This technique will no doubt be further tested and fine-tuned, so it may become even more likely that a couple willing to go through this procedure can have a boy. But at this stage, there are several significant problems with this particular approach for the average person.

First of all, there are only a limited number of centers in

the United States that offer this service. The expense and trouble of traveling to those spots will undoubtedly deter the vast majority of couples.

But an even more important point of resistance will probably be the idea of conceiving by artificial insemination. Somehow, if a couple can rely on a sex-selection technique that is available in their own bedrooms, that seems more acceptable and *natural* than going the test-tube route. Many people have an instinctive reaction to the idea of conceiving via laboratory processing. They can't quite explain their feelings—but they know they just don't like the idea.

Others *can* explain how they feel. And they do so readily in such terms as these: "This smacks too much of genetic engineering." Or "How do you know treating and manipulating the sperm outside the body won't cause birth defects?" Or "This approach is just going too far for me to be able to reconcile it with my religious faith." As a result of such negative attitudes, many researchers conducting fertility and sex-selection experiments that require artificial insemination have run into great difficulty getting volunteers.

So the inconvenience or a sense of an unnatural or mechanistic approach to intercourse has deterred couples from turning in droves to this gender-selection technique—as well as to those previously mentioned. If spouses have a basic fertility problem, they are more likely to cast aside their reservations. But for most people, the question of selecting the sex of a baby just doesn't rise to the same level of importance as the question of whether they can conceive at all.

But there is a more acceptable and palatable scientific hope for preconception sex selection on the horizon—in the form of influencing your baby's gender through a perfectly natural diet.

5. **THE DIET APPROACH TO PRECONCEPTION SEX SELECTION.** It's long been suspected that there may be a connection between what a woman eats and the sex of the

baby she conceives. We've already seen numerous examples of this belief in the folklore relating to methods of gender determination.

In her book *Boy or Girl?*, Elizabeth Whelan details a few attempts by medical doctors during the past century to find a key to preconception sex selection in diet. These include Dr. Leopold Schenk's 1898 book, *The Determination of Sex*, in which he told women who wanted sons to go on a high-protein, low-carbohydrate diet, and those who desired daughters to try sweets and other carbohydrates.

Most of these early theories, when taken by themselves, certainly don't stand up to scientific scrutiny. But some recent research with both animals and humans into the possible relationship of diet and gender determination indicates that the ancients may have been on the right track after all. In fact, some of the findings suggest that a woman's food intake can influence her future offspring's sex with about as high a chance of success as the older, more complicated, and less convenient scientific approaches we've already discussed.

In other words, it seems that by altering her diet—within the normal bounds of good nutrition and demands for tasty foods—a woman may be able to greatly increase the odds that she'll have a boy or a girl when she conceives. But this subject requires more than a few short paragraphs to understand, so let's move on now to a fuller discussion in the next chapter.

Can You Diet Your Way to a Boy or a Girl? 4

THERE HAS BEEN an assumption since ancient times that a woman's diet can influence whether she conceives a boy or a girl. In the last fifty years, scientific studies, with both animals and human beings, have shown that these traditions of folklore have a solid basis in fact.

Some significant research began to be reported in Germany in the 1930s by a Dr. Curt Herbst, who had been studying the process of sex determination in a marine worm, the bonellia. He and subsequent researchers found that sex in these and other primitive marine creatures is influenced by varying the ratio of potassium to calcium and magnesium in the surrounding environment. Specifically, if you increase the potassium and lower the calcium and magnesium, you get more males. And if you lower the potassium and raise the level of calcium and magnesium, more females are the result.

In a later series of experiments, Dr. Joseph Stolkowski, of the University of Pierre and Marie Curie in Paris, found that the same principle applies to cattle. He increased the potassium/calcium-magnesium ratio by having the animals lick sodium chloride lumps (ordinary table salt), which increased the concentrations of both sodium and potassium in body tissue. Those animals that were given extra sodium gave birth to more males, and those given less sodium conceived more females.

The next and in many ways the most significant development in this research occurred when a doctor named Jacques Lorrain, from the department of gynecology and obstetrics at the Sacre-Coeur Hospital in Montreal, got quite excited about Stolkowski's findings. He decided to collaborate with Stolkowski to see if the same approach that had worked with worms and cattle might also work with human beings.

As with the primitive marine worms and the cattle, the basic scientific hypothesis they wanted to test here was whether increasing the ratio of potassium to calcium and magnesium in women's food would produce more males. Conversely, they wanted to see if decreasing the potassium and increasing the calcium and magnesium would result in more girl babies.

The main technique they used was similar to what Stolkowski had done in his experiments with cattle: They increased the sodium intake of those women who wanted boys.

More sodium, in other words, would mean more potassium "ions" (or electrically charged potassium atoms) in body tissue. More potassium, in turn, would supposedly enhance the likelihood that boys would be conceived. To aid in the buildup of potassium ions, a decision was also made to add more potassium to the diet and to restrict the amounts of calcium and magnesium.

Restricting these latter two minerals further enhances the movement of potassium into the body's tissues because the ions of all three (potassium, calcium, and magnesium) tend to "compete" with one another. The ions that are present in the highest concentrations are usually the ones that are taken up by the body tissue in the largest quantities.

The opposite approach was chosen for women who wanted female babies. Salt would be severely restricted in their diet. To strengthen the chance that a girl would be conceived, the dietary intake of calcium and magnesium was increased, and the intake of potassium was reduced. These dietary maneuvers were supposed to diminish the concentration of potassium ions in body tissue even further.

After considerable transatlantic personal communications during the 1970s, the two doctors conducted a series of studies with 281 women, ages nineteen to thirty-nine, in Europe and North America. Their findings, which have been published in articles in the *International Journal of Gynaecology and Obstetrics*, showed that more than 80 percent of the women participating in a controlled diet program could conceive a child of the desired sex.

Specifically, here's the technique they employed: Taking the potassium-ion theory that had worked in the animal experiments, Lorrain and Stolkowski put the women who wanted boys on a diet high in salt and potassium, and those who desired girls on a low-salt, low-potassium, and high-calcium diet. The food regimen began four to six weeks before any attempts were made to conceive, and the participants were asked to continue with the diet until they conceived or until six months had elapsed. If they hadn't conceived at the end of six months, they were supposed to consult with a doctor. The husbands were also asked to follow the diet, primarily to give their wives moral support.

For those who wanted a boy, the menus for this experimental diet were designed to provide a daily intake of 297 milligrams of calcium, 135 milligrams of magnesium, 5,000 milligrams of sodium, and 3,873.5 milligrams of potassium. To be certain they got enough potassium, the doctors prescribed two 600-milligram tablets daily of potassium chloride (called "Slow-K").

The specifics of the "girl diet" were quite different. These women were asked to consume daily foods containing 1,528 milligrams of calcium, 254 milligrams of magnesium, 675 milligrams of sodium, and 2,947 milligrams of potassium. This regimen was to be supplemented each day with a 500-milligram tablet of calcium and also with vitamin D.

Lorrain and Stolkowski, by the way, in one of their articles in the *International Journal of Gynaecology and Obstetrics*, warned that there may be "contraindications," or dangers, in their diet for women with certain health problems. For example, the highly salted boy diet may be bad for hypertension (high blood pressure). The two doctors also reported that four women on the salty boy diet dropped out because they began to suffer from water retention.

On the other hand, the high-calcium, low-salt diet for girls may create problems of a different kind. Women on this program were cautioned if they had tendencies toward excessive nervousness, kidney problems, or overabundant amounts of calcium in their blood.

Of the 281 women who started the program, only 21 dropped out—either because they felt the system was too strict, because they went off the diet before they got pregnant, or because they developed negative reactions of some sort. Of the 224 women who finished Lorrain's part of the study, 181—or 81 percent—gave birth to a child of the gender they had wanted. Of the 36 women under Stolkowski's guidance, 31 were successful in conceiving a baby of the desired sex, for an 86 percent success rate.

Why does this diet approach to gender selection apparently work?

At this point, nobody seems to know for certain. Both Lorrain and Stolkowski have their pet theories, but any explanations must, for the time being, remain in the realm of speculation.

One *possible* reason for the success of the experiments may be that the diets are causing the woman's egg to become more receptive to one kind of sperm than another. In other words, the high-salt diet may make the egg more receptive to Y (male) sperm, while the high-calcium, low-salt diet may aid the action of the X (female) sperm.

Another possible explanation that has been offered for the impact of the diet is that since the husbands were encouraged to follow it as well as the wives, the food intake may have had some decisive impact on their sperm, rather than on the women's eggs.

Ultimately, though, how a diet can influence the gender of a baby is not understood. For one thing, the manipulation of sodium, potassium, calcium, and magnesium intake within normal dietary ranges is known to have little effect on the *overall* concentrations of these elements in the body. The reason for this is that the body has many mechanisms for stabilizing these concentrations in response to ordinary variations in what a person eats. Any attempt to change these overall concentrations by severely unbalancing the diet would involve grave health risks—but with the Lorrain-Stolkowski approach, we're not talking about any such radical approach to eating habits.

So we have to look for an answer in another direction, and here is one of the most reasonable explanations that has been offered:

It may be possible that the concentration of certain ions in *specific* body tissues can be altered. This is so because tissues are made up of cells that have structures called "receptors." These receptors may be attached to the surface of the cell membrane or imbedded within it. The activity of many of these receptors is influenced by changes in the ionic concentrations of the surrounding bodily environment.

For example, large concentrations of sodium ions in the body tend to "excite" receptors. In their excited state, the receptors will grab on to almost any kind of ion that "interests" them. Receptors that will accept potassium, by the way, will also accept calcium and magnesium. So if calcium and magnesium ions are significantly outnumbered by potassium ions, the receptors are much more likely to grab on to the potassium

Thus, by increasing sodium and potassium in the diet, the

local environment in which sperm meets egg may be richer in potassium—and thereby enhance the fertilization of the egg by the male Y-bearing sperm. The child in this case is more likely to be a boy.

The opposite approach to eating may lead to an opposite result: Low concentrations of sodium ions in the body tend to diminish receptor activity. By also reducing the amount of potassium and increasing the amounts of calcium and magnesium in the diet, the ions that are grabbed by the receptors will tend to be those of calcium and magnesium.

In this case, the region where fertilization takes place may be poorer in potassium, thereby giving the female X-bearing sperm a better chance of penetrating the egg. Thus, the child would more likely be a girl.

Until more research is done, however, *any* attempt to explain how varying the ratio of potassium to calcium and magnesium in body tissue can affect a baby's gender has to remain purely speculative. All we can say for sure, given the evidence we now have, is that what a woman eats in the weeks immediately prior to conception does play an important role in determining the sex of her baby. In other words, by consciously adhering to a well-planned preconception diet, a woman can increase her chances of conceiving a baby of the sex she desires.

The results can be dramatic for women who have decided to try to conceive a child of a certain sex by altering their diets. For example, a June 1981 issue of the French newspaper *France Dimanche* reported that a young French woman who was on a diet formulated by Dr. Stolkowski found "victory at the end of the road. She wanted a boy; she had a boy."

"The happiness of my marriage was at stake," the woman reportedly said. "My husband already had three girls from a previous marriage, and he wanted an heir very badly. When he told me that he wished to have a child by me, he said, 'I want a boy—it is a son that I want.' For me it was a difficult time. I was already thirty-four and I was afraid I was too old to have a child."

The young woman even confided: "His desire to have a son was so strong that I was afraid that he would look for another woman outside our marriage who would bear him a son."

With this kind of pressure bearing down on her, the wife turned to the diet approach to gender control, which she had heard about through her job as a teacher of dietetics. She went on a high-salt, low-calcium diet prescribed by the medical center doing the study, and a few months later, she became pregnant.

But it hadn't been easy for her—primarily because of the way she had been required to change her eating habits. The diet the center put her on included things she didn't like, such as bananas and corned beef. Also, she had to avoid things she did like, such as many commercial desserts, milk chocolate, and especially cheese.

"I love all kinds of cheese," she said longingly. "I made up my mind to have an all-cheese meal right after conception."

When she finally became pregnant, it was an enormous relief for her to return to her old eating habits. And most important of all, when the long-awaited baby finally arrived, this young French woman and her husband were ecstatic because it was, indeed, a boy.

So there is a growing body of scientific evidence—and personal testimonials—that diet can make a difference in whether your child will be a boy or a girl. But this conclusion shouldn't be so surprising in light of certain other information that has been accumulated over the years.

For one thing, there is the interesting phenomenon of the variation of sex ratios at birth in different geographical, cultural, and ethnic groups. In the United States, the normal ratio of boys to girls at birth is 105 to 100—and that ratio tends to represent an overall norm or average throughout the world.

But in earlier historical periods there were some reports of much more dramatic differences in the boy-girl ratio in certain cultures. And even today, according to current demographic studies, this ratio varies rather consistently from nation to nation (though as we've said, the international *average* tends to be about 105:100, boys to girls).

For example, in a study reported by W. T. Russell in the 1936 *Journal of Hygiene,* Greece and Korea had the highest boy-to-girl ratios in the world, with 113 newborn boys for every 100 girls. England and Japan, on the other hand, reported the lowest ratios in these early studies, with about 104 boy babies to every 100 girl babies.

In earlier studies conducted in predominantly Jewish populations, the ratio of males to females was usually found to be quite high. For example, an investigation into Jewish birth ratios in the Austrian empire during the years 1904, 1907, and 1910 revealed a male-to-female sex ratio at birth of more than 109 boys to every 100 girls.

Current statistical studies also show variations of the boy-girl ratios at birth, even though the differences often aren't as pronounced as those reported by the earlier investigations. One good source for this information is the 1975 *Demographic Yearbook* published by the United Nations, which contains a "special topic" on natality statistics. This volume provides raw data showing how many boys and how many girls were born in many nations and colonies each year between 1956 and 1975.

To get a better picture of the sex-ratio issue, we have calculated from this data the average boy-to-girl birth ratios for several nations during the 1956–75 period. For example, we found that the United States, between 1956 and 1975, maintained an average boy-to-girl ratio of 105.1 newborn boys to every 100 newborn girls. This finding was approximately the same ratio that had always been assumed for the United States and came as no surprise.

Greece, on the other hand, had an average birth ratio of 107 boys to 100 girls during the 1956–75 period—down somewhat from the previously reported ratio of 113 to 100, but still higher than those of the United States and many other nations that consistently remain closer to the 105:100 norm.

Hong Kong—the only available listing in this UN study for a predominantly Chinese population (since information about Red China and Taiwan was not available)—also had a relatively high ratio of 107.1 boys to 100 girls over the nearly twenty years that these statistics were tabulated.

Japan, which was listed in one earlier study as having one of the lowest boy-girl birth ratios in the world, was relatively high in the UN survey with 106.4 boys for every 100 girls. The other "low-boy" country in those earlier studies was England, with a reported ratio of 104.3 boys born for every 100 girls. But in the UN findings, the United Kingdom was up to 106 boys for every 100 girls.

Israel, which has one of the most clearly identifiable Jewish populations in the world, had an average ratio of 106.2 boys to every 100 girls. This is a figure somewhat lower than the 109:100 ratio that was found in the investigations in the early part of this century in the Austrian empire, but it's still higher than the international norm.

Now, can we make any generalizations from these sex ratios that may help us understand a little better the role of diet in determining a child's gender?

First of all, a few cautionary comments: It's obvious that even though there are variations in the most recent sex ratios we've cited, those variations are still rather slight—say on the order of about 1 to 2 percent more boys in some countries than in others.

Perhaps the reason that the sex ratios are lower in some of the newer studies is simply that modern statistical methods are more advanced and accurate than they were in the early part of this century.

Another important factor may be that diets have changed significantly in many nations around the world as a result of wider dissemination of knowledge about nutrition. Also, as more countries have developed their technology and raised their standard of living, they have developed more sophisticated transportation systems which have facilitated the export and import of foreign foods. This whole process of modernization has brought many of the divergent peoples of the world closer together—and has enhanced the similarities in the way they work, think, dress, and eat.

But even though the differences in the boy-to-girl baby ratios in the countries we've selected are rather small, they still do represent *consistent* differences over nearly two decades. And they pose an important question: Why should women in some countries regularly give birth to proportionately more boys or girls than women in other countries?

No one has been able to come up with a definitive answer to this question. But there is speculation that differences in diet may be a likely explanation.

For example, as you'll see when you look through the sample menus for the "diet to conceive a boy" in chapter six, there are a number of dishes that involve Greek, Chinese, or Jewish kosher types of cooking. Of course, it's hard to generalize about any nation's eating traditions because there are always so many variations from individual to individual. But there is a *tendency* in ethnic Greek and Chinese families to serve foods that are relatively high in potassium and salt.

As for Jewish foods, the many Jews who are ethnically assimilated into other cultures tend to eat just like anyone in those cultures, and their eating habits have little to teach us in our investigation. On the other hand, Orthodox Jews, who follow strict kosher menus, have a very distinctive style of eating—and many of their dishes are quite similar to the kinds of foods that scientific researchers have found tend to produce more boys than girls.

For example, shellfish, like oysters and shrimp, are forbidden in kosher menus. And these same foods, which tend to be high in calcium, are associated in some recent scientific research (when they are boiled and their water is eliminated) with foods that tend to produce females rather than males. In contrast, in all the available sex-ratio studies for newborn babies in Jewish cultures, there tend to be more boys than average.

For example, as we've just seen, the boy-girl ratio for Israel, which was 106.2 boy babies for every 100 girl babies born between 1956 and 1975, is higher than the ratio in the United States and many other countries. This difference may be due in part to the kosher tradition among many Jews who live in Israel.

On the other hand, as any sociologist or political scientist knows, the religiously observant Orthodox Jews in Israel are in a minority, and there are also many residents of Israel of non-Jewish extraction. So perhaps the boy-to-girl ratio is no higher there because the "boy-diet" food intake of the Orthodox Jews has been "diluted" by the presence of so many who feel free to eat a broader range of foods.

This question of the relationship of a population's diet to sex determination will probably never be satisfactorily resolved until some controlled studies are done on the eating habits in villages or towns with an exceptionally high or low boy-to-girl baby ratio. Until that happens, we can only talk in terms of possibilities and "maybe's." But the facts, as they now stand, tend to point toward a nutritional explanation of the differences in the ratios.

Several interesting observations on these national birth ratios have been offered by a professional nutritionist with broad international experience, Dorcas Demasio. Demasio received her B.S. in nutrition and dietetics from New York University and her M.S. in nutrition and dietetic health from Columbia University. She also holds a United Nations diploma in international nutrition and food science from the University of Wageningen, in the Netherlands.

From her considerable academic study and practical experience dealing with food habits in a wide variety of countries, Demasio has concluded that there is a definite correlation between (*a*) the average diets in Greece, Chinese communities like Hong Kong, and Jewish kosher communities and (*b*) the "boy diets" and "girl diets" that scientists like Jacques Lorrain and Joseph Stolkowski have tested on human beings.

In other words, the typical daily menus in those three cultures, which have tended to produce more boy babies than the average, are *weighted* in favor of foods relatively high in salt and potassium and low in calcium and magnesium. This is not to say that the average woman in those countries has the *best* or *ideal* diet to produce a boy, but just that the general types of foods she eats probably increase the odds that she'll have a male baby.

At this point, then, the jury is still out on this question of the meaning of the varying boy-girl ratios at birth in different cultures. But the evidence continues to pile up in favor of a dietary interpretation.

As a result, we've tentatively concluded that there is some causal relationship between *(a)* the typical foods that women in those cultures eat before they become pregnant and *(b)* the variations in sex ratios in different countries and cultures.

We also believe further research will show that those cultures producing the most boys at birth will be the same ones having typical diets that are relatively high in salt and potassium and low in calcium and magnesium. Conversely, the cultures with more girl babies at birth will be those with typical diets higher in calcium and magnesium and lower in potassium and salt.

Finally, in addition to these considerations about the significance of different sex ratios at birth, it's also interesting to note a few points about one of the first topics we covered in this book—the traditional folk methods to control whether you'll have a boy or a girl.

Persistent folk beliefs and traditions are often relegated automatically to the status of silly superstitions by later, more scientific ages. And it's certainly true that some of the old wives' tales that encouraged women of earlier eras to eat certain things in order to conceive a boy and other things to conceive a girl may have been completely off base.

But before we laugh too hard, let's examine a few of these

substances to see if their mineral and nutritional composition fits into what we've been learning about the influence diet has on gender control.

■ *Oysters:* As we saw in the first chapter, there's a tradition in Ghana, on the western coast of Africa, that eating boiled oysters without the saltwater solution will enhance a woman's chance of bearing a female baby. In support of this notion, there are numerous stories natives of this country can tell about women who followed a heavy oyster diet and then had a passel of girls.

One native of Ghana actually told us, "I know a woman who loved to have many daughters. So she ate raw oysters regularly over a period of years, and the first five children she and her husband had were girls."

So what exactly is in an oyster that may have this influence on gender?

According to publications of the U.S. Department of Agriculture and other scientific sources on nutrition, a half cup of raw oysters contains relatively large amounts of calcium (approximately 113 to 152 milligrams) and iron (approximately 6.6 to 8.1 milligrams). Other minerals present in oysters include potassium (120-plus milligrams), phosphorus (150-plus milligrams), and sodium (80-plus milligrams).

When we use the term *relatively large amounts,* we're referring to the amount of a given mineral or other substance in the food in relation to the amounts that would be consumed daily in an average, healthy diet. For example, most nutrition experts would suggest that the average daily adult diet should contain 800 milligrams of calcium, while the average for potassium may range much higher—perhaps from 2,000 to 6,000 milligrams daily. So even though the *absolute* number of milligrams of, say, calcium (113-plus) in the oysters might be less than the absolute number of potassium (120-plus milligrams), the amount of the calcium relative to what is present in the average diet is much greater. (In other words, 113 milligrams represents a relatively high percentage of the 800-milligram daily requirement for calcium, while 120 milligrams of potassium represents a relatively small percentage of the daily potassium intake of 2,000 to 6,000.) So what can we conclude from all this?

Here's one possibility: If the nutritional composition of oysters has any significance at all in determining the gender of a female child, either iron or calcium or both may well be substances that play a role in the process. The word *calcium* should ring a bell with you by now because that mineral is emerging as one of the key substances that should be in a woman's diet in quantity if she wants to conceive a girl.

■ *Fish and red meats cooked in salty solutions:* Various cultures around the world have included these two items in folk diets that are supposed to produce a boy baby.

One aspect of the nutritional breakdown for these foods is quite obvious: High amounts of sodium would have to be present simply because of the use of significant amounts of salt in cooking, as well as natural amounts of sodium present in the foods themselves.

In addition, most foods in the fish and red-meat categories would contain relatively high amounts of potassium and low amounts of calcium. For example, 3.5 ounces of broiled halibut contain about 540 milligrams of potassium, and the same amount of baked flounder has nearly 600 milligrams of potassium. On the other hand, both of these fish—as well as most other fish—are quite low in calcium.

Most beef dishes containing 3-ounce servings have between 300 and 400 milligrams of potassium and small amounts of calcium.

So you can see that this particular folk tradition is, once again, quite consistent with recent scientific studies on gender control in that the foods recommended are high in sodium and potassium and low in calcium.

■ *Sweets and desserts:* There is a widespread folk tradition that if a woman wants to have a girl she should eat a lot of sweets and desserts. Now it may be that this idea arose merely from the notion that girls are "sugar and spice and everything nice." But there has been a strong persistence of this tradition over the years, and the idea was incorporated seriously into a number of early books on dietary theories of gender control.

It's rather difficult to analyze as vague a category as "sweets and desserts" because there is such a wide range of food values in this category. Most pies, for example, contain rather large amounts of sodium—say, from about 300 to 600 milligrams. And pies like apple, cherry, lemon, mince, and pumpkin contain relatively small amounts of potassium, but they are also generally rather low in calcium as well. So if we wanted to focus on *these* particular sweets and desserts, they would come closer to fitting into a boy diet rather than a girl diet.

On the other hand, desserts with a milk base, like puddings, custards, and ice creams, tend to be high in calcium and low in potassium and sodium—and that formula, of course, is quite consistent with what we've come to know about a likely girl diet.

■ *Lion's blood and wine:* As was mentioned earlier, this combination, along with intercourse under a full moon, was supposed during the Middle Ages to result in a boy baby. But the tradition involving just the drink actually goes back even further, to ancient Rome, where it was also supposed to be drunk as a potion to produce a male child.

An analysis of lion's blood isn't particularly encouraging, though if the blood is allowed to stand long enough to clot, the watery portion, or serum, does have a substantial number of "cations" of potassium. A cation, by the way, is a positively charged atom of a certain element—in this case, potassium.

Table wine, on the other hand, has a substantial amount of potassium—about 100 milligrams in a half cup. In fact, except for a small amount of iron, potassium is practically the only substance of any nutritional value in a glass of wine.

■ *Cowpeas.* Cowpeas, you'll recall, were both thrown across a local road and also consumed in substantial quantities in certain rural American communities by those young women who wanted boy babies.

As it happens, these women were anticipating recent scientific findings, because cowpeas—especially immature ones—are one of the best boy foods around. They contain very little calcium and are loaded with potassium. If a woman can stand to eat two-thirds of a cup of them raw, she'll get 541 milligrams of potassium. And even if she cooks them, she'll still get 303 milligrams.

We could continue on and on with these descriptions of folk diets that are supposed to influence a baby's gender, but the main point has been made: Many of the old wives' formulas were actually harbingers of what has been revealed by scientific research.

Of course, not all the folk foods fit precisely into what modern researchers are discovering about gender diets. But there are still an amazing number of correlations that can perhaps explain why so many of these folk formulas lasted for such long periods of time. In short, our ancestors happened to hit on at least part of the right dietary formula. And that may mean that the women who followed these formulas had a greater degree of success in influencing their babies' gender than those who ignored the diet approach altogether.

This, then, represents the scientific case for the validity of a preconception gender-control diet—with a few words of support thrown in from sex-ratio statistics and folklore traditions. The weight of the evidence seems to indicate that if you go on a diet consistent with these findings, you'll greatly increase your chances of having a boy or a girl.

But from a medical point of view, is it a good idea to go on such a diet? Or, to put it more bluntly, are these proposed boy and girl diets safe? Let's turn to these issues before we get any deeper into specific diet programs.

Some Red Lights for Women on Special Diets 5

As WE'VE SEEN in the previous chapter, the diet that is most likely to work in influencing the gender of your next child involves adjustments of four minerals in your daily food intake: potassium, sodium, calcium, and magnesium.

If you want the best chance of conceiving a boy, you should increase the intake of sodium and potassium and decrease the amounts of calcium and magnesium. On the other hand, if you want a girl, you do the opposite: Decrease the sodium and potassium and increase the calcium and magnesium.

But can you make the required adjustments in your daily food menus and still maintain an acceptable level of health?

To answer this question, it's necessary first of all to evaluate the present state of your own health—and that means having a physical examination. As has been mentioned, this book isn't designed to be a substitute for your physician. Before you follow either of the diet programs in this book, you should consult your doctor. Second, it's important to understand a little more about what those four minerals actually do in your body, and what the consequences are likely to be if their amounts are varied in the human system.

So now let's examine each of these four substances in some detail so that we can see what role they characteristically play in your personal health—and also what inferences we can draw about them for a preconception gender diet.

1. **SODIUM.** Sodium, or salt, is found in copious quantities in the average diet of Western nations. In fact, even though some nutrition tables list the daily "requirement" of sodium at only 500 milligrams, the average American diet has more like 2,000 to 6,000 milligrams.

Too much sodium in the diet may aggravate a tendency toward hypertension (high blood pressure), so before you go on any diet that is high in salt, be sure you know the status of your blood pressure.

On the other hand, some writers on nutrition in pregnancy have become concerned about too little salt in the diets of pregnant women. Gail and Tom Brewer, in their book, *What Every Pregnant Woman Should Know*, stress the importance of extra salt as the blood volume of the pregnant woman increases and the placenta, the lifeline of the fetus, develops. But most obstetricians and nutritionists seem to feel that this need for extra salt really becomes important only in the second and third trimesters of pregnancy, as the growing baby gets bigger and puts more nutritional demands on the mother's system.

As far as the requirements of a preconception gender diet are concerned, there appear to be no problems with either low- or high-salt food programs. For example, in the study done by Drs. Lorrain and Stolkowski, the "girl diet" was set at 675 milligrams of sodium daily. It would be possible to go even lower, down to 500 milligrams, and still remain within what most nutritionists regard as the healthy range.

For the highly salted "boy diet," these researchers established a daily sodium intake of 5,000 milligrams daily. This is well within the usual daily consumption of 2,000 to 6,000 milligrams that nutritionists expect. (We want to stress once more, however, that anyone with a personal or family history of hypertension should be very careful about increasing salt intake.)

2. **POTASSIUM.** Most dieticians seem to feel that a reasonably balanced Western diet will provide enough potassium without it being necessary to keep precise track of how much is consumed each day. The general view is that there is no definite daily requirement for potassium, though most nutrition manuals list 2,000 to 4,000 milligrams as the amount contained in the "usual diet."

Too little potassium in the system may result in "hypokalemia," an unusual condition resulting most often from special therapies and drugs that act as diuretics and increase a person's urine flow. Too much potassium is also relatively unusual and is frequently triggered by some other major physical problem, like acute kidney failure.

For the kinds of diets that are associated with preconception gender control, these radical variations in the body's potassium don't seem to be a problem. The Lorrain-Stolkowski potassium diet for conceiving a girl was 2,947 milligrams, and the amount for a boy was 3,873.5 (with a prescribed daily supplement of 1,200 milligrams of potassium chloride). The girl-diet amount was well within the usual range of a healthy diet. The boy-diet allocation, even though it was somewhat higher than the normal daily requirement, certainly doesn't seem to have been excessive in light of the current literature on the subject.

3. **CALCIUM.** Most nutritionists believe that the average daily calcium requirement for adults is 800 milligrams, and for pregnant and nursing women, 1,200 milligrams.

Calcium is important in causing hardness of teeth and bones and helping blood coagulation. It also plays a role in many other bodily functions, such as facilitating muscle contraction and relaxation and inducing smooth heart action. Too little calcium may result in "hypocalcemia," which may be accompanied by a deficiency in vitamin D and lead to such problems as bone demineralization, fragile bones, and even heart arrest. In pregnant women, especially in the last two trimesters, there may also be a negative impact on the development of the fetus.

On the other hand, those having too much calcium, or "hypercalcemia," may show such signs as physical weakness, fatigue, sleepiness, or kidney and digestive problems like vomiting or constipation.

So how do the gender diets measure up in light of these requirements?

The girl diet used by Lorrain and Stolkowski included 1,528 milligrams of calcium daily, with a daily tablet supplement of 500 milligrams, for a grand total of 2,028 milligrams. For those having problems with too much calcium in their system, this regimen might be too much. So it's important for women with any tendency toward hypercalcemia to keep in close touch with a doctor. Also, those with high cholesterol blood readings may want to stress low-fat or no-fat dairy products in their menus. For most people, though, this amount of calcium would present no problem.

The Lorrain-Stolkowski boy diet, however, may cause some difficulties for certain people. At a suggested rate of 297 milligrams daily, the calcium amounts are significantly below what is regarded by most nutritionists to be the minimum daily requirement, 800 milligrams. On the other hand, the doctors and nutritionists we approached indicated that not enough is known about this area of nutrition for them to be able to say with any certainty what the precise impact of this low calcium intake would be on the average person.

But one thing does seem fairly certain: Any negative impact from a low level of calcium in the diet would probably occur over a relatively long period of time—at least many months and perhaps several years. So the normal, healthy woman who went on one of these diets for up to six months probably wouldn't experience any difficulties.

4. **MAGNESIUM.** Some studies of proper mineral balance in human diets have concluded that the average adult needs from 250 to 300 milligrams of magnesium each day. Most nutrition texts, as well as recommendations of the National Research Council, set the daily requirement a little higher, at 300 milligrams for women and 350 for men.

People who get too little magnesium over a long period of time may develop problems related to their cardiovascular system, their kidneys, and their nervous and muscular systems. A deficiency of magnesium in the human body may create symptoms like excessive irritability, anxiety, and hypertension. Alcoholics and individuals with very serious kidney diseases are among those most likely to experience a magnesium deficiency.

Too much magnesium may also be present in the systems of people with kidney failure. In this case, the symptoms include lethargy and difficulty in breathing.

The amount of magnesium prescribed in the girl diets that have been medically tested is somewhat low at 254 milligrams, but it is still well within acceptable limits according to reliable medical studies. On the other hand, the magnesium amount in the boy diet used by Lorrain and Stolkowski, 135 milligrams daily, is lower than the minimum requirement suggested by most nutritionists. But even those who oppose going on a diet of this type concede that any deleterious effects would probably be the result of a long-term, cumulative deficiency.

So in light of this nutritional analysis, what can we conclude about the safety of a preconception gender diet?

First of all, there is no problem at all with the dietary formula to conceive a girl, including the mineral balances used in the Lorrain-Stolkowski studies.

On the other hand, the boy diet, as it has been presented by Lorrain and Stolkowski, does present us with a few questions—especially with respect to the low daily amounts of calcium and magnesium. Certainly the low amounts of these substances wouldn't be at all acceptable during the second and third trimesters of pregnancy because of the increased needs of the mother-to-be and her growing fetus. Hence, once a woman on a preconception gender-selection diet finds out she's pregnant, she should go on a regular pregnancy diet.

But with these words of caution in mind, a nonpregnant woman or a man whose diet is balanced in every other respect and who is in good health should be able to go on a low-calcium, low-magnesium diet for a limited duration—say for several months—and experience no ill effects. In any case, people on *any* special diet should stay in close contact with their physicians and undergo regular checkups to be sure that no exceptional changes are occurring in their bodies.

Now you know something about how special diets can improve your chances to conceive either a boy or a girl. And you also have a good idea of the important nutritional considerations involved in such diets.

So the time has arrived for a practical look at how you can go on such a diet yourself. In the following pages, we have sifted through all the available information and, in close collaboration with a professional nutritionist, formulated two original sixty-day model diets. The first is for those women who want to conceive a boy, and the second is for those who want a girl.

Diet A: Diet to Conceive a Boy

6

IN LIGHT OF the research involving animals and human beings—and also with the key food-oriented folk traditions in mind—we collaborated with professional nutritionist Dorcas Demasio, whose credentials have been described in chapter 4, to put together a "sixty-day diet to conceive a boy." A comparable diet for a girl will be included in the next chapter.

But first, let us emphasize once again the importance of caution: It's essential that individuals first check with a physician to be certain that possible health problems—like hypertension or kidney difficulties—would not prevent them from following either of these diets.

Also, remember that at this stage in the development of this technique it's by no means certain you'll conceive a child of the desired sex, even if you follow these diets to the letter. Scientific research suggests that you'll greatly improve your chances to have a boy or a girl. But there's still the possibility that you'll have a boy even if you were expecting a girl, and vice versa. So if you're hoping for a girl, you should still be open to a boy—and be prepared to love either!

These diets, while they follow the guidelines discussed in the previous two chapters, have also been designed with an eye to maintaining a healthy, balanced food intake. The suggested daily consumption of calories has been held at about 1,800. If you follow these suggested menus closely, it will probably be unnecessary for you to supplement the diets with potassium or calcium tablets, as some experts in this area have suggested. As we've indicated, a trained nutritionist has put these diets together to provide all the basic foods you need for a healthy diet, and her work has been carefully checked by another professional nutritionist.

In addition, in view of recent findings about the possibly deleterious impact on the fetus of caffeine and alcohol ingested by a pregnant woman, we have omitted these substances from the menus. Our assumption here is that a woman could be pregnant and still be on these gender diets for a brief period of time before she becomes aware of her condition. Of course, as we've said before, as soon as a woman finds out she is pregnant, she should go off the gender-selection diet and begin a regular pregnancy diet under the guidance of her physician.

Now, a few specifics about our suggested "boy diet."

You'll note that the foods in the sample menus are high in salt and low in calcium. You may *not* see, unless you're a trained nutritionist, that they are also relatively high in potassium and low in magnesium.

The average daily mineral ranges for the boy diet are: 5,000 to 6,000 milligrams of sodium; 4,000 to 5,000 milligrams of potassium; 250 to 400 milligrams of calcium; and 120 to 200 milligrams of magnesium.

These specifications have some interesting implications for those whose taste buds draw them to certain home-cooked or restaurant-prepared ethnic dishes. For example, Demasio suggests that those on the boy diet might find some possible dishes in

Mexican, Chinese, Korean, Greek, Jewish kosher, and "soul" or American southern cooking. Also—and those concerned about problems with American dietary habits may cringe at this point—many of the salty "fast foods," like hamburgers, fried fish, and french fries, may meet the boy diet requirements.

Even though there are certain nutritional guidelines you should follow to give these diets the best chance of success, there is a fairly wide variety of available dishes that may suit even the most discriminating of palates—especially for the boy diet. Furthermore, if you want to create your own menus, here's a way you can go about it:

The menus on each of the two sixty-day diets are *interchangeable* to the extent that you can substitute items in major food categories for one another (e.g., vegetables for vegetables, meats for meats, etc.) and still retain approximately the same food values. Also, it's possible to exchange entire meals for one another (e.g., a lunch on one day for a lunch on the next). And of course, if you'd prefer to eat a meal that is listed as a lunch on any given day for a dinner on that day, and eat the dinner as your lunch, that's fine, too. Also, if you'd like to include foods that aren't on these suggested daily menus, we've prepared an appendix at the back of this book that shows you how to substitute still other equivalent dishes and still keep your food intake consistent with the gender diet.

Obviously, many times you may find yourself in a situation where you can't prepare these menus in the comfort of your own home—as when you have to go out to work. In those situations, we suggest that if it's convenient you try "brown-bagging it" by making one of the suggested cold dishes, such as a sandwich, at home and then bringing that with you.

Sometimes this approach will be impossible, and for those cases, when you have to order from a restaurant menu, here are some guidelines:

- Order raw fruits and vegetables because they contain more

potassium than the comparable amounts of cooked, canned, or frozen fruits and vegetables.

■ Fats tend to be some of the foods lowest in potassium, and refined cereals are the next lowest, though many cereals tend to be high in sodium content. It's important to check the labels on cereals to be sure about what you're getting.

■ High-protein foods, such as steaks and roasts, tend to be richer in potassium content.

■ Avoid milk and milk products, like custards.

We've based both our suggested boy and girl diets on a sixty-day cycle. There are thirty separate menus, which should be used for the first thirty days and then repeated for the next thirty days. During the first thirty days you're on the diet, you should continue to use some form of birth control. After thirty days, you can begin to try to conceive. Be sure to stay on the diet until pregnancy is confirmed. We recommend that you have your physician give you regular checkups while you're on this regimen. You should abandon the diet at once if you notice any abnormalities in your usual bodily functions. And in any case, it's best to let your system "rest" by going off the diet if you haven't conceived within six months.

And here's one final, important point we want to make: We suggest that both the prospective mother and father go on this diet. Why? Because any diet—even one as tasty as these are—is hard to maintain if the person on it doesn't have some moral support at times. And there is no better support for a diet than a "buddy system," whereby one person can rely on the other if temptations to eat forbidden foods get too great.

Also, by joining the woman, the man will gain a greater sense of participation—a feeling that will likely carry over into pregnancy and later parental responsibilities as well. A decision to go on a diet together presupposes a fair amount of conversation and personal interaction, and that can only mean more meaningful communication—and a deeper love relationship.

If you don't know how to prepare some of the dishes mentioned in this chapter and the next, check with chapter 8, which includes some of the more complex recipes for both the boy and the girl diets. An asterisk appears next to each dish for which a recipe is provided. If you need further help, you can consult any popular, comprehensive cookbook and use the recipes there—so long as you keep in mind that salt can be used in the boy diet, but should be avoided for the girl diet.

Now, with these basic principles in mind, let's turn our attention to some actual menus for a possible "boy diet."

DAYS 1 AND 31

BREAKFAST:

   8 oz orange juice
   2 sausage links
   1 soft-cooked egg
   1 slice white toast
   1 tsp butter
   weak tea, black decaffeinated coffee

LUNCH:

   3 oz veal and pepper*
   1/2 cup Spanish rice* (can be bought in store)
   1/2 cup green beans, preferably raw or only slightly
      cooked
   1 slice white bread
   1 tsp butter or margarine
   1/2 cup orange sherbet
   black decaffeinated coffee

DINNER:

   3 oz corned tongue with gravy (buy it prepared and heat)
   1 parsley potato (boiled, with parsley decoration)
   1/2 cup mashed squash
   1 slice white bread
   1 tsp margarine or butter
   1 banana
   black decaffeinated coffee

SNACK:

   8 oz grapefruit juice
   24 dates (1 cup)

DAYS 2 AND 32

BREAKFAST:

8 oz prune juice
3 slices bacon
1 soft-cooked egg
1 slice white toast
1 tsp butter or jelly
weak tea, black decaffeinated coffee with lemon

LUNCH:

1/2 cup chicken matzo-ball soup (buy it prepared in store)
4 oz pink salmon*
1/2 cup rice
1/2 cup cooked chopped broccoli (buy frozen)
1/2 cup coleslaw
1/2 cup canned peaches
black decaffeinated coffee with lemon

DINNER:

1 cup vegetarian vegetable soup (buy it prepared)
3 oz tuna fish salad (with lettuce and tomatoes)
beet salad (cut one beet in pieces and boil for 15-20 min.)
1 slice white bread
1 tsp margarine or butter
herbal tea, black decaffeinated coffee

SNACK:

8 oz prune juice
2 large chestnuts (roasted) (3 small)

DAYS 3 AND 33

BREAKFAST:

8 oz orange juice
3 slices bacon
1 soft-cooked egg
1 slice white toast
1 tsp butter or jelly
herbal tea, black decaffeinated coffee

LUNCH:

1 open club sandwich with sausage links (lettuce, tomato, and sausage links on white bread)
lettuce and tomato salad with any dressing
1/2 cup strawberries
herbal tea, black decaffeinated coffee

DINNER:

8 oz orange juice
3 oz baked pork chops
1/2 cup cabbage
2/3 cup fruit cocktail
herbal tea, black decaffeinated coffee

SNACK:

8 oz grapefruit juice
3/4 cup raisins

DAYS 4 AND 34

BREAKFAST:

8 oz orange juice
3 slices bacon
1 soft-boiled egg
1 slice white toast
1 tsp butter or jelly
herbal tea, black decaffeinated coffee with lemon

LUNCH:

8 oz tomato juice
3 oz chicken breast (fried in corn oil)
1/2 cup rice
1/2 cup cooked kidney beans
lettuce and tomato salad, any dressing
2 tsp mayonnaise
1 slice white bread
1 tsp butter
herbal tea, black decaffeinated coffee

DINNER:

3 oz roast beef, sirloin
1 oz beef broth gravy
1/2 cup rice
1/2 cup carrots, preferably raw
3/4 cup tossed lettuce salad with 1 tsp french dressing
1 slice white bread
1 tsp butter
1 banana
herbal tea, black decaffeinated coffee with lemon

SNACK:

1 cup apricots (fresh, dried, or canned)

DAYS 5 AND 35

BREAKFAST:

8 oz orange juice
3 slices bacon
1 soft-boiled egg
1 slice white toast
1 tsp jelly or butter
black decaffeinated coffee with lemon

LUNCH:

8 oz tomato juice
3 oz hamburger with garnish (decorative garnish can be vegetables such as green pepper or onion, fried in butter)
1/2 cup macaroni salad
1 slice white bread
1 tsp butter
1 cup apricots
black decaffeinated coffee

DINNER:

8 oz grapefruit juice
3 franks and 3/4 cup sauerkraut
1/2 cup raw celery
1/10 cut average size watermelon
black decaffeinated coffee

SNACK:

8 oz prune juice
2 oatmeal cookies

DAYS 6 AND 36

BREAKFAST:

8 oz grapefruit juice
3 slices bacon
1 soft-cooked egg
1 slice white toast
1 tsp margarine or jelly
black decaffeinated coffee

LUNCH:

3 oz corned beef and cabbage with mustard
1 boiled potato
1/2 cup pumpkin* (boiled for 15-20 min.)
1 slice white bread
1 tsp margarine
1/2 cantaloupe
black decaffeinated coffee

DINNER:

3 oz sauteed liver*
1 mashed potato
1/2 cup wax beans, slightly cooked
1/2 cup fiesta coleslaw*
1 slice white bread
1 tsp butter or margarine
1 banana
black decaffeinated coffee

SNACK:

1 cup prunes

DAYS 7 AND 37

BREAKFAST:

    8 oz blended juice—orange or grapefruit (as sold in store)
    3 slices bacon
    1 soft-cooked egg
    1 slice white toast
    1 tsp butter or jelly
    black decaffeinated coffee

LUNCH:

    8 oz tomato juice
    3 oz roast turkey
    1/2 cup mashed sweet potato
    1/2 cup asparagus
    1 slice white bread
    1 tsp butter
    1/2 cup orange sherbet
    herbal tea, black decaffeinated coffee

DINNER:

    3 oz boiled chicken
    1 tsp butter
    1 baked potato
    1/2 cup cooked cabbage
    lettuce and tomato salad, dressing
    1/2 grapefruit
    herbal tea, black decaffeinated coffee

SNACK:

    1 banana

DAYS 8 AND 38

BREAKFAST:

    8 oz prune juice
    2 sausage links
    1 soft-boiled egg
    1 slice white toast
    1 tsp butter or jelly
    black decaffeinated coffee

LUNCH:

    4 oz Hawaiian chicken*
    1/2 cup sweet potato and apple (in cans, follow label)
    1/2 cup cooked (buy frozen) chopped broccoli
    1 slice white bread
    1 tsp butter
    1 cup canned apricots
    black decaffeinated coffee with lemon

DINNER:

    4 oz beef potpie (buy prepared)
    1/2 cup raw cucumbers
    1 slice white bread
    1 tsp margarine
    1 banana
    black decaffeinated coffee

SNACK:

    1/2 cup cherries
    8 oz orange juice

DAYS 9 AND 39

BREAKFAST:

8 oz orange juice
3 slices bacon
1 soft-boiled egg
1 slice white bread
1 tsp butter
black decaffeinated coffee

LUNCH:

8 oz tomato juice
3 oz Yankee pot roast*
1/2 cup parsley potato
1/2 cup cut green beans and mushrooms
1 slice white bread
1 tsp butter
1 banana
black decaffeinated coffee

DINNER:

8 oz tomato juice
3 oz broiled veal
1 baked potato
1/2 cup sliced carrots, preferably raw
1 soft roll
1 tsp butter
1/2 cup pears
black decaffeinated coffee, weak tea

SNACK:

8 oz grapefruit juice
2 oatmeal cookies

DAYS 10 AND 40

BREAKFAST:

8 oz orange juice
2 sausage links
1 soft-boiled egg
1 slice white toast
1 tsp butter or jelly
black decaffeinated coffee

LUNCH:

8 oz tomato juice
3 oz fried chicken
1/2 cup french fries
lettuce and tomato with any salad dressing
1 banana
black decaffeinated coffee

DINNER:

1 cup stewed prunes (canned)
3 oz pepper steak with fried mushrooms
celery and tomato with any salad dressing
1 slice white bread
1 tsp butter
black decaffeinated coffee

SNACK:

8 oz grapefruit juice
1/2 cup strawberries

DAYS 11 AND 41

BREAKFAST:

8 oz orange juice
2 slices bacon
1 soft-cooked egg
1 slice white toast
1 tsp butter
black decaffeinated coffee

LUNCH:

3 oz cornish hen* with mushroom stuffing
1 tbl cranberry sauce
1 sweet potato
1/2 cup mushrooms (fried*, or boiled for 15-20 min.)
1 slice white bread
1 tsp butter
1 banana
black decaffeinated coffee

DINNER:

3 oz beef stew
1/2 cup plain rice
tomato salad with mayonnaise dressing
1 slice white bread
1 tsp margarine
black decaffeinated coffee with lemon

SNACK:

8 oz grapefruit juice
1 cup dates

DAYS 12 AND 42

BREAKFAST:

    8 oz orange juice
    3 slices bacon
    1 soft-cooked egg
    1 slice white toast
    1 tsp butter or margarine
    weak tea, black decaffeinated coffee

LUNCH:

    8 oz tomato juice
    3 oz rolled fish* with lemon
    1/2 cup beans supreme*
    1/2 cup fiesta coleslaw*
    1 slice white bread
    1 tsp butter or margarine
    1 slice strawberry pie
    black decaffeinated coffee

DINNER:

    3 oz veal, sliced on club roll
    1/2 cup carrot and raisin salad (sold in store)
    1 banana
    black decaffeinated coffee

SNACK:

    1 cup apricots
    8 oz grapefruit juice

DAYS 13 AND 43

BREAKFAST:

8 oz grapefruit juice
3 slices bacon
1 soft-cooked egg
1 slice white toast
1 tsp butter
black decaffeinated coffee, herbal tea

LUNCH:

8 oz tomato juice
3 oz broiled steak
1 baked potato
1 tsp butter
1/2 cup celery and lettuce salad with oil and vinegar dressing
1 banana
black decaffeinated coffee, herbal tea

DINNER:

5 oz spaghetti and meatballs in tomato sauce
2 slices tomato on 1/2 cup lettuce
1 fresh orange
herbal tea, black decaffeinated coffee

SNACK:

8 oz grapefruit juice
1 slice strawberry pie (store bought)

DAYS 14 AND 44

BREAKFAST:

8 oz grapefruit juice
3 slices bacon
1 soft-cooked egg
1 slice white toast
1 tsp butter
black decaffeinated coffee with lemon

LUNCH:

3 oz roast brisket
1/2 cup parsley potato
1/2 cup cooked chopped broccoli (buy frozen)
1 slice white bread
1 tsp butter
1 banana
black decaffeinated coffee

DINNER:

8 oz tomato juice
3 oz broiled chicken livers
1/2 cup baked lima beans
1 baked potato
1 cup prunes
black decaffeinated coffee with lemon

SNACK:

2 large chestnuts, roasted (3 small)
8 oz orange juice

DAYS 15 AND 45

BREAKFAST:

8 oz orange juice
3 slices bacon
1 soft-boiled egg
1 slice white toast
1 tsp butter or jelly
black decaffeinated coffee

LUNCH:

4 oz chicken fricassee*
1/2 cup Spanish rice*
1/2 cup fresh chopped celery
1 sliced tomato on lettuce, oil and vinegar
1 slice white bread
1 tsp butter
1 banana
black decaffeinated coffee

DINNER:

3 oz Yankee pot roast*
1 baked potato
10 fried mushrooms*
1 tomato and lettuce with french dressing
1 slice white bread
1 tsp butter
1 banana
black decaffeinated coffee

SNACK:

8 oz tomato juice
2 oatmeal cookies

DAYS 16 AND 46

BREAKFAST:

8 oz grapefruit juice
3 slices bacon
1 soft-cooked egg
1 slice white toast
1 tsp margarine or butter or jelly
black decaffeinated coffee, weak tea

LUNCH:

8 oz tomato juice
3 oz pepper steak
1/2 cup egg barley (store-bought cereal, in box)
1/2 cup sliced beets
1 banana
1 slice white bread
1 tsp margarine
black decaffeinated coffee

DINNER:

4 oz Spanish omelet
1/2 cup hashed brown potatoes
1 slice white bread
1 tsp butter
1/2 cup fresh apple and celery salad with oil and vinegar dressing
10 strawberries (1/2 cup)
black decaffeinated coffee

SNACK:

5 medium-size figs
8 oz grapefruit juice

DAYS 17 AND 47

BREAKFAST:

    8 oz orange juice
    3 slices bacon
    1 soft-boiled egg
    1 slice white toast
    1 tsp butter or jelly
    black decaffeinated coffee with lemon

LUNCH:

    4 oz franks and beans
    sliced tomato salad with oil and vinegar dressing
    1/2 cup chopped fresh celery
    1 slice white bread
    1 tsp butter
    1 banana
    black decaffeinated coffee

DINNER:

    1 ham sandwich with mustard
    cucumber and tomato salad
    2/3 cup fresh fruit cup (canned)
    black decaffeinated coffee

SNACK:

    8 oz grapefruit juice
    1 banana

DAYS 18 AND 48

BREAKFAST:

8 oz orange juice
3 slices bacon
1 soft-cooked egg
1 slice white toast
1 tsp butter
decaffeinated coffee with lemon

LUNCH:

8 oz tomato juice
3 oz bologna sandwich on white bread with lettuce and mustard
1/2 cup chopped celery
1 banana
black decaffeinated coffee

DINNER:

1 cup vegetable soup (canned)
3 oz broiled hamburger steak
1 baked potato
1/2 cup pickled beets
1 slice white bread
1 tsp margarine or butter
black decaffeinated coffee

SNACK:

1/2 cup frozen or fresh strawberries
2 sandwich biscuits

DAYS 19 AND 49

BREAKFAST:

8 oz grapefruit juice
3 slices bacon
1 soft-cooked egg
1 slice white toast
1 tsp butter
black decaffeinated coffee, weak tea

LUNCH:

4 oz roast fresh ham with gravy (bought already cooked, served cold or heated)
1 baked sweet potato
1/2 cup baked lima beans
1 banana
black decaffeinated coffee

DINNER:

8 oz tomato juice
4 oz boiled veal
1/2 cup cooked broccoli
lettuce and tomato salad with oil and vinegar dressing
1/2 cup pears
black decaffeinated coffee

SNACK:

1 cup pitted cut dates
8 oz grapefruit juice

DAYS 20 AND 50

BREAKFAST:

8 oz orange juice
3 slices bacon
1 soft-cooked egg
1 slice white toast
1 tsp margarine
black decaffeinated coffee

LUNCH:

3 oz corned beef hash
1/2 cup mixed vegetables, carrots and peas only slightly cooked
tossed tomato and lettuce salad with oil and vinegar dressing
1 cup stewed prunes
black decaffeinated coffee

DINNER:

8 oz tomato juice
4 oz sauerbraten
3/4 cup red cabbage
1 banana
black decaffeinated coffee

SNACK:

3/4 cup raisins
8 oz grapefruit juice

DAYS 21 AND 51

BREAKFAST:

    8 oz orange juice
    3 slices bacon
    1 soft-cooked egg
    1 slice white toast
    1 tsp butter
    black decaffeinated coffee, weak tea

LUNCH:

    3 sausage links on a bun with canned relish
    3/4 cup sauerkraut
    1/2 cup potato salad
    1 cup apricots
    black decaffeinated coffee

DINNER:

    8 oz tomato juice
    3 oz roast brisket
    1 baked potato
    1/2 cup baked lima beans
    1 cup stewed prunes
    black decaffeinated coffee

SNACK:

    3/4 cup raisins
    8 oz grapefruit juice

DAYS 22 AND 52

BREAKFAST:

    8 oz grapefruit juice
    3 slices bacon
    1 soft-cooked egg
    1 slice white toast
    1 tsp butter
    black decaffeinated coffee

LUNCH:

    8 oz tomato juice
    4 oz potted Swiss steak*
    1/2 cup mashed potatoes
    1/2 cup baked lima beans
    1 banana
    black decaffeinated coffee

DINNER:

    sardine salad with garnish*
    2 slices tomato, lettuce and celery salad with oil and vinegar dressing
    1 roll
    1 tsp butter
    1 cup grapefruit sections
    black decaffeinated coffee

SNACK:

    8 oz grapefruit juice
    3/4 cup raisins

DAYS 23 AND 53

BREAKFAST:

    8 oz orange juice
    3 slices bacon
    1 soft-cooked egg
    1 slice white toast
    1 tsp butter
    black decaffeinated coffee, weak tea

LUNCH:

    4 oz honey-drip chicken*
    1/2 cup parsley potatoes
    1/2 cup beets in orange sauce
    1 slice white bread
    1 tsp margarine or butter
    1 banana
    black decaffeinated coffee

DINNER:

    8 oz tomato juice
    3 oz roast beef
    1/2 cup rice
    1 cup prunes
    1 slice white bread
    1 tsp butter or margarine
    1 cup dates
    black decaffeinated coffee

SNACK:

    8 oz grapefruit juice
    2 cookies homemade

DAYS 24 AND 54

BREAKFAST:

8 oz grapefruit juice
1 soft-cooked egg
1 slice white toast
1 tsp margarine or jelly
black decaffeinated coffee

LUNCH:

3 oz roast lamb
1 tsp mint jelly
1/2 cup mashed potatoes
1/2 cup carrot pennies, preferably raw
1 slice white bread
1 tsp margarine or butter
1 banana
black decaffeinated coffee

DINNER:

8 oz tomato juice
4 oz boiled chicken
1 oz gravy from chicken
1 cup egg barley
1 slice white bread
1 tsp margarine
1/2 cup cherries
black decaffeinated coffee

SNACK:

8 oz orange juice
10 strawberries (1/2 cup)

DAYS 25 AND 55

BREAKFAST:

    8 oz grapefruit juice
    3 slices bacon
    1 soft-cooked egg
    1 slice white toast
    1 tsp butter
    black decaffeinated coffee

LUNCH:

    4 oz salmon salad cold plate*
    1/2 cup celery
    1 slice white bread
    1 tsp butter or margarine
    black decaffeinated coffee

DINNER:

    4 oz sliced loin of pork with gravy
    1 baked apple
    1/2 cup fresh artichokes
    1 banana
    black decaffeinated coffee

SNACK:

    1 orange

DAYS 26 AND 56

BREAKFAST:

8 oz blended juice—orange and grapefruit
1 soft-cooked egg
1 slice white toast
1 tsp butter or jelly
black decaffeinated coffee

LUNCH:

3 oz roast chicken
1 oz brown gravy
1 baked potato
1/2 cup cooked broccoli (buy frozen)
1 slice white bread
1 tsp butter
10 strawberries (1/2 cup)
black decaffeinated coffee

DINNER:

3 oz pepper steak
1 oz gravy
1/2 cup noodles
1/2 cup tossed salad, including lettuce, green peppers, tomatoes, with oil and vinegar dressing
1 banana
black decaffeinated coffee

SNACK:

8 oz grapefruit juice
3/4 cup raisins

DAYS 27 AND 57

BREAKFAST:

8 oz orange juice
3 slices bacon
1 soft-cooked egg
1 slice white toast
1 tsp butter or jelly
black decaffeinated coffee

LUNCH:

4 oz fried chicken
1 tsp butter
1/2 cup rice
1/2 cup baked lima beans
1 sliced tomato on lettuce
1 slice white bread
1 tsp butter
1 banana
black decaffeinated coffee

DINNER:

3 oz roast beef, sirloin
1 oz beef broth gravy
1 large baked potato
1/2 cup carrots, preferably raw
1/2 cup tossed salad, with lettuce, tomatoes, and green peppers, with 1 tsp french dressing
1 slice white bread
1 tsp butter
black decaffeinated coffee

SNACK:

8 oz tomato juice
2 oatmeal cookies

DAYS 28 AND 58

BREAKFAST:

    8 oz orange juice
    3 slices bacon
    1 soft-cooked egg
    1 slice white toast
    1 tsp butter or jelly
    black decaffeinated coffee

LUNCH:

    8 oz tomato juice
    3 oz short ribs*
    1 oz gravy
    1/2 cup potatoes
    1/2 cup peas
    1 slice white bread
    1 tsp margarine
    1/2 cup pear halves
    black decaffeinated coffee

DINNER:

    3 oz boiled chicken with coleslaw
    1/2 cup baked lima beans
    1/2 cup lettuce and tomatoes with any dressing
    1 slice white bread
    1 tsp margarine
    1/2 cup peaches
    black decaffeinated coffee

SNACK:

    1 banana

DAYS 29 AND 59

BREAKFAST:

8 oz orange juice
2 sausage links
1 soft-cooked egg
1 slice white toast
1 tsp butter
black decaffeinated coffee

LUNCH:

8 oz tomato juice
3 oz rolled fish* with lemon
1/2 cup beans supreme*
1/2 cup fiesta coleslaw*
1 slice white bread
1 tsp butter or margarine
10 strawberries (1/2 cup)
black decaffeinated coffee

DINNER:

4 oz Salisbury steak with fried mushrooms*
1/2 cup hashed brown potatoes
1/2 cup buttered peas
1 banana
black decaffeinated coffee

SNACK:

3/4 cup dates or raisins
8 oz grapefruit juice

DAYS 30 AND 60

BREAKFAST:

8 oz prune juice
3 slices bacon
1 soft-cooked egg
1 slice white toast
1 tsp butter or jelly
black decaffeinated coffee

LUNCH:

4 oz fried chicken
1 baked sweet potato with skin
1/2 cup cooked chopped broccoli (buy frozen)
1 slice white bread
1 tsp butter or margarine
1 cup apricots
black decaffeinated coffee

DINNER:

4 oz baked salmon
1/2 cup fresh cucumbers, mixed with 4 slices tomatoes
    and lettuce with any dressing
1 slice white bread
1 tsp margarine
1/2 cup pears
black decaffeinated coffee

SNACK:

8 oz prune juice
2 large chestnuts (3 small), roasted

Diet B: Diet to Conceive a Girl

7

THIS "DIET FOR A GIRL BABY," which was also prepared in collaboration with our professional nutritionist, Dorcas Demasio, is quite different from the regimen for a boy—but it's been prepared with an eye to making it just as palatable and tasty.

One major distinguishing characteristic of the girl diet is that it's very low in salt. Many nutritionists would argue that this is a good thing because Americans eat far too much salt anyway—with possible negative physical repercussions like hypertension.

On the other hand, as we've already mentioned previously, some nutritionists do get concerned if salt intake is too low during pregnancy. This becomes an issue especially during the second and third trimesters, when the blood volume is increasing, the placenta is developing, and other biological changes that require extra salt are occurring in the bodies of the woman and the fetus.

As with the boy diet, the girl diet is based on a sixty-day cycle. There are thirty separate menus, which should be used for the first thirty days and then repeated for the next thirty days. During the first thirty days you're on the diet, you should continue to use some form of birth control. After thirty days, you can begin to try to conceive. Be sure to stay on the diet until pregnancy is confirmed. We recommend that you have your physician give you regular checkups while you're on this regimen. You should abandon the diet at once if you notice any abnormalities in your usual bodily functions. And in any case, it's best to let your system "rest" by going off the diet if you haven't conceived within six months.

We also recommend that a woman go off this diet as soon as she learns she's pregnant and start a pregnancy diet under the supervision of her physician. In this way, she will be getting all the nutrients she needs for herself and her growing baby as early as possible in the first trimester.

The average daily mineral ranges for the girl diet are as follows: sodium, 700 to 1,000 milligrams; potassium, 2,500 to 3,500 milligrams; calcium, 1,2000 to 1,800 milligrams; and magnesium, 200 to 300 milligrams.

Another special feature of the girl diet is that there is much more room for sweets than on the boy diet. But one limitation here is that the desserts and other sugary items must, generally speaking, be *homemade*. The reason for this is that most commercial desserts contain too much salt for them to fit within the girl menus.

With these considerations in mind, nutritionist Demasio has also offered several other suggestions for women who are interested in trying to give birth to a girl through this food-intake technique:

- Don't use water softeners for drinking water around your home—they introduce too much salt into the water.
- Eliminate all commercial ice cream and sherbets from your diet—again, too much salt.
- Avoid using baking soda or baking powder in your cooking.

- Read labels of all packed foods, as well as of on-the-shelf medicines like laxatives, carefully for sodium or salt content.
- Acceptable drinks for the girl diet include: ginger ale, cranberry juice, grape juice, pineapple juice, cranapple juice, and apricot nectar. Weak decaffeinated coffee (preferably with milk) is also all right.
- If you like carbonated beverages, limit yourself to 8 ounces for the entire day.
- Avoid commercial chocolate syrup, instant cocoa, and alcoholic beverages—all contain too much salt for the diet.
- Take one-half of a 100-milligram Vitamin C tablet each day, as indicated in the menus, to supplement your daily needs.

These general principles also apply when you're eating out in restaurants. And as with the boy diet, you're free to substitute the meals or foods in like categories (vegetables for vegetables, etc.) for one another. Just be sure that you stick to the foods listed on the menus. The appendix in this book also shows you how to substitute some equivalent dishes and still keep food intake consistent with the diet.

Now, with these guidelines in mind, let's turn to the sixty-day series of menus for the girl diet. As in the boy diet, an asterisk appears next to each dish for which a recipe is given in the following chapter. The term *salt-free*, which appears with many items, means two things. For items such as baked potatoes or eggs, no salt should be added in cooking or at the table. For items such as margarine or bread, it means a salt-free product should be purchased.

DAYS 1 AND 31

BREAKFAST:

1/2 100-mg vitamin C tablet
4 oz grape juice
1 salt-free soft-boiled egg
1 slice salt-free toast
1 tsp salt-free margarine
1 tsp honey
4 oz milk
other drinks: see chapter introduction

LUNCH:

2 oz salt-free broiled steak
1 oz salt-free gravy
1 salt-free small potato
1/2 cup salt-free green beans
1 slice salt-free bread
1 tsp salt-free butter
1 slice salt-free homemade apple pie*
4 oz milk
other drinks: see chapter introduction

DINNER:

2 oz salt-free roast chicken
1 oz salt-free gravy
1/2 cup salt-free white rice
1/2 cup salt-free canned carrots
lettuce, salt-free salad dressing
1/2 cup custard*
4 oz milk
other drinks: see chapter introduction

SNACK:

8 oz plain yogurt with 1/3 cup canned diced pineapple

DAYS 2 AND 32

BREAKFAST:

    1/2 100-mg vitamin C tablet
    4 oz apple juice
    1 salt-free poached egg
    1 slice salt-free toast
    1 tsp salt-free butter
    4 oz milk
    other drinks: see chapter introduction, add 1 tsp sugar if desired

LUNCH:

    2 oz salt-free Salisbury steak
    lettuce, salt-free salad dressing
    1 salt-free small boiled potato
    1 salt-free roll
    1 tsp salt-free margarine
    1/10 cut fresh watermelon
    4 oz milk
    other drinks: see chapter introduction

DINNER:

    2 oz rolled fish* with egg sauce*, salt-free
    1/2 cup salt-free Spanish rice*
    lettuce, salt-free salad dressing
    1 slice salt-free bread
    1 tsp salt-free butter
    1/2 cup canned pears without juice
    4 oz milk
    other drinks: see chapter introduction

SNACK:

    2 salt-free cookies
    3 oz piece salt-free cheese

DAYS 3 AND 33

BREAKFAST:

1/2 100-mg vitamin C tablet
4 oz grape juice
1 salt-free poached egg
1 slice salt-free toast
1 tsp salt-free butter
4 oz milk
other drinks: see chapter introduction

LUNCH:

2 oz salt-free pepper steak
lettuce and cucumber salad, salt-free salad dressing
1 slice salt-free bread
1 tsp salt-free butter
1/2 cup salt-free custard*
4 oz milk
other drinks: see chapter introduction

DINNER:

1 salt-free small baked potato
1/2 cup salt-free asparagus soufflé*
1/2 cup salt-free canned carrots
1 salt-free soft roll
1/2 cup canned peaches without juice
4 oz milk
other drinks: see chapter introduction

SNACK:

6 oz milk
2 salt-free homemade cookies

DAYS 4 AND 34

BREAKFAST:

1/2 100-mg vitamin C tablet
4 oz grape juice
1 salt-free poached egg
1 slice salt-free toast
1 tsp salt-free butter
4 oz milk
other drinks: see chapter introduction

LUNCH:
1 cup salt-free cottage cheese
1/2 cup canned peaches and pears without juice
lettuce and cucumber salad, salt-free salad dressing
1/10 cut honeydew melon (in season)
drinks: see chapter introduction

DINNER:
2 oz salt-free baked fish
1 salt-free small boiled potato
1/2 cup sliced cooked carrots
1/2 cup canned pineapple without juice
drinks: see chapter introduction

SNACK:
6 oz milk
1 salt-free homemade pastry (salt-free pastry also available in stores—read labels)

DAYS 5 AND 35

BREAKFAST:

1/2 100-mg vitamin C tablet
4 oz apple juice
1 salt-free soft-boiled egg
1 slice salt-free toast
1 tsp salt-free margarine
4 oz milk
other drinks: see chapter introduction, add 1 tsp sugar if desired

LUNCH:

2 oz salt-free baked chicken
1/2 cup salt-free rice
1/2 cup salt-free green beans
1 slice salt-free bread
1 tsp salt-free butter
1/2 cup peach halves
4 oz milk
other drinks: see chapter introduction

DINNER:

2 oz salt-free Salisbury steak
1/2 cup mixed cooked vegetables, unsalted carrots and peas (no spinach)
1/2 cup salt-free mashed potato
1 slice salt-free bread
1 tsp salt-free butter
1 papaya
4 oz milk
other drinks: see chapter introduction

SNACK:

5 almonds
4 oz milk

DAYS 6 AND 36

BREAKFAST:

1/2 100-mg vitamin C tablet
4 oz grape juice
1 salt-free soft-cooked egg
1 slice salt-free toast
1 tsp salt-free butter
drinks: see chapter introduction, add 1 tsp sugar if desired

LUNCH:

2 oz salt-free roast lamb
1 oz mint jelly
1 salt-free small boiled potato
1/2 cup carrot pennies
1 slice salt-free bread
1 tsp salt-free butter
1/2 cup canned peaches (without liquid)
4 oz milk
other drinks: see chapter introduction

DINNER:

2 oz salt-free baked fish
lettuce wedge
1/2 cup salt-free plain rice
1 slice salt-free bread
1 tsp salt-free butter
1/2 cup salt-free custard* (except chocolate)
4 oz milk
other drinks: see chapter introduction

SNACK:

8 oz salt-free strawberry yogurt
4 oz milk

DAYS 7 AND 37

BREAKFAST:

1/2 100-mg vitamin C tablet
4 oz grape juice
1 salt-free soft-cooked egg
1 slice salt-free toast
1 tsp salt-free margarine or butter
1 tsp honey to sweeten decaffeinated coffee
4 oz milk
other drinks: see chapter introduction

LUNCH:

2 oz salt-free sliced lamb
1 oz salt-free gravy
1 salt-free boiled potato
1/2 cup sliced carrots
1 slice salt-free bread
1 tsp salt-free butter
1/10 cut watermelon
4 oz milk
other drinks: see chapter introduction

DINNER:

2 oz salt-free boiled chicken leg
1/2 cup salt-free white rice
1/2 cup salt-free wax beans
1 slice salt-free bread
1 tsp salt-free butter
1/2 cup gelatin dessert
4 oz milk
other drinks: see chapter introduction

SNACK:

4 oz milk
1/2 cup canned peaches without juice

DAYS 8 AND 38

BREAKFAST:

1/2 100-mg vitamin C tablet
4 oz grape juice
1 salt-free poached egg
1 slice salt-free toast
1 tsp salt-free butter
4 oz milk
other drinks: see chapter introduction

LUNCH:

2 oz salt-free veal
1 salt-free small boiled potato
1/2 cup salt-free green beans
1 slice salt-free bread
1 tsp salt-free butter or margarine
1/2 cup canned pineapple, without juice
drinks: see chapter introduction

DINNER:

2 oz salt-free liver*
1/2 cup sliced fresh cucumbers
1 salt-free small baked potato
1 slice salt-free bread
1 tsp salt-free margarine
1/2 cup canned pears without juice
4 oz milk
other drinks: see chapter introduction

SNACK:

1/2 cup plain yogurt
8 oz milk

DAYS 9 AND 39

BREAKFAST:

1/2 100-mg vitamin C tablet
4 oz apple juice
1 salt-free poached egg
1 slice salt-free toast
1 tsp salt-free butter
4 oz milk
other drinks: see chapter introduction

LUNCH:

2 oz salt-free boiled turkey
1 salt-free small boiled potato
1/2 cup lettuce, salt-free salad dressing
1/2 cup canned pears without juice
1 slice salt-free bread
1 tsp salt-free butter
4 oz milk
other drinks: see chapter introduction

DINNER:

2 oz salt-free roast beef
1/2 cup salt-free parsley potatoes
1/2 cup chopped asparagus
1/2 cup canned pear halves without juice
4 oz milk
other drinks: see chapter introduction

SNACK:

6 oz milk
1 slice salt-free cheese
2 wafers of rusks (hard crackers)

DAYS 10 AND 40

BREAKFAST:

1/2 100-mg vitamin C tablet
4 oz apple juice
1 salt-free poached egg
1 slice salt-free toast
1 tsp salt-free butter
4 oz milk
other drinks: see chapter introduction, add 1 tsp sugar if desired

LUNCH:

2 oz salt-free braised short ribs*
1 oz salt-free gravy (juice from cooked meat)
1 salt-free small baked potato
1/2 cup canned pears without juice
1/2 cup sliced cucumbers
1 slice salt-free bread
1 tsp salt-free margarine
4 oz milk
other drinks: see chapter introduction

DINNER:

2 oz salt-free baked fish fillet
1/4 cup mashed potato
1/2 cup salt-free green beans
1 slice salt-free bread
1 tsp salt-free butter
1/2 cup applesauce
4 oz milk
other drinks: see chapter introduction

SNACK:

1 3-oz piece salt-free cheese
two rusks

DAYS 11 AND 41

BREAKFAST:

1/2 100-mg vitamin C tablet
4 oz grape juice
1 salt-free soft-cooked egg
1 tsp salt-free margarine or butter
4 oz milk
other drinks: see chapter introduction

LUNCH:

2 oz Yankee pot roast*, salt-free
1 salt-free small parsley potato
1/2 cup salt-free green beans
1/6 cut honeydew melon
1 slice salt-free bread
1 tsp salt-free margarine
4 oz milk
other drinks: see chapter introduction

DINNER:

1 salt-free small baked potato
1/2 cup asparagus soufflé*, salt-free
1/2 cup sliced carrots (boiled), salt-free
1 salt-free roll
1 tsp salt-free margarine
1/2 cup canned peaches without juice
4 oz milk
other drinks: see chapter introduction

SNACK:

1 salt-free homemade pastry
6 oz milk

DAYS 12 AND 42

BREAKFAST:

1/2 100-mg vitamin C tablet
4 oz apple juice
1 salt-free poached egg
1 slice salt-free toast
1 tsp salt-free butter or margarine
4 oz milk
other drinks: see chapter introduction

LUNCH:

2 oz plain salt-free chicken
1/2 cup egg barley
1/2 cup sliced carrots
1 slice salt-free bread
1 tsp salt-free margarine or butter
1/2 cup canned peaches without juice
4 oz milk
other drinks: see chapter introduction

DINNER:

2 oz salt-free plain omelet
1/2 cup salt-free mashed potatoes
1 cup salt-free frozen cauliflower (boiled)
1/2 cup canned peaches without juice
1 slice salt-free bread
1 tsp salt-free butter
4 oz milk
other drinks: see chapter introduction

SNACK:

6 oz milk
2 salt-free wafers

DAYS 13 AND 43

BREAKFAST:

1/2 100-mg vitamin C tablet
4 oz grape juice
1 salt-free soft-cooked egg
1 slice salt-free toast
1 tsp salt-free butter
4 oz milk
other drinks: see chapter introduction

LUNCH:

2 oz salt-free roast beef
1 oz salt-free gravy
1 salt-free boiled potato
lettuce wedge
1 slice salt-free bread
1 tsp salt-free butter
1/2 cup canned pineapple without juice
4 oz milk
other drinks: see chapter introduction

DINNER:

2 oz salt-free sliced chicken
1/2 cup salt-free steamed rice
1/2 cup sliced carrots
1 slice salt-free bread
1 tsp salt-free butter
1/2 cup canned peaches without juice
drinks: see chapter introduction

SNACK:

6 oz milk
1/2 cup frozen strawberries

Days 14 AND 44

BREAKFAST:

1/2 100-mg vitamin C tablet
4 oz apple juice
1 salt-free soft-cooked egg
1 slice salt-free toast
1 tsp salt-free margarine or butter
4 oz milk
other drinks: see chapter introduction

LUNCH:

2 oz salt-free sirloin steak
1/2 cup salt-free green beans
1 salt-free small baked potato
1 tsp salt-free butter or margarine
1/2 cup canned pineapple without juice
4 oz milk
other drinks: see chapter introduction

DINNER:

2 oz salt-free liver*
1/2 cup salt-free plain rice
1/2 cup sliced cooked carrots
1 slice salt-free bread
1 tsp salt-free butter or margarine
1/2 cup frozen strawberries
4 oz milk
other drinks: see chapter introduction

SNACK:

6 oz milk
2 tsp salt-free peanuts

DAYS 15 AND 45

BREAKFAST:

1/2 100-mg vitamin C tablet
4 oz grape juice
1 salt-free soft-cooked egg
1 slice salt-free toast
1 tsp salt-free butter or margarine
4 oz milk
other drinks: see chapter introduction

LUNCH:

2 oz salt-free veal
1/2 cup salt-free plain rice
1/2 cup diced carrots
1/2 cup custard
1 slice salt-free bread
1 tsp salt-free butter or margarine
drinks: see chapter introduction

DINNER:

2 oz salt-free liver*
1 salt-free small boiled potato
1/2 cup salt-free green beans
1 slice salt-free bread
1 tsp salt-free butter or margarine
1/2 cup canned pears without juice
4 oz milk
other drinks: see chapter introduction

SNACK:

6 oz milk
1 salt-free homemade pastry

DAYS 16 AND 46

BREAKFAST:

1/2 100-mg vitamin C tablet
4 oz apple juice
1 salt-free soft-cooked egg
1 slice salt-free toast
1 tsp salt-free butter or margarine
4 oz milk
other drinks: see chapter introduction

LUNCH:

2 oz sliced salt-free lamb
1/2 cup sliced salt-free zucchini
1 small salt-free boiled potato
1 slice salt-free bread
1 tsp salt-free butter or margarine
1/2 cup sliced canned peaches without juice
drinks: see chapter introduction

DINNER:

2 oz salt-free rolled fish* with lemon wedge
1/2 cup salt-free mashed potato
1/2 cup salt-free cooked carrots
1 slice salt-free bread
1 tsp salt-free butter or margarine
1/10 cut salt-free homemade apple pie*
4 oz milk
other drinks: see chapter introduction

SNACK:

1/2 salt-free tuna sandwich
6 oz milk

DAYS 17 AND 47

BREAKFAST:

1/2 100-mg vitamin C tablet
4 oz grape juice
1 salt-free poached egg
1 slice salt-free toast
1 tsp salt-free margarine or butter
4 oz milk
other drinks: see chapter introduction

LUNCH:

2 oz salt-free steak
2 oz salt-free gravy
1/2 cup salt-free mashed potato
lettuce wedge
1/2 cup cucumber
1 slice salt-free bread
1 tsp salt-free butter
1/2 cup gelatin dessert
4 oz milk
other drinks: see chapter introduction

DINNER:

4 oz salt-free baked macaroni and cottage cheese
1/2 cup salt-free peas
1 slice salt-free bread
1 tsp salt-free margarine
1/2 cut melon
4 oz milk
other drinks: see chapter introduction

SNACK:

6 oz milk
salt-free homemade strawberry pie*

DAYS 18 AND 48

BREAKFAST:

    1/2 100-mg vitamin C tablet
    4 oz apple juice
    1 salt-free soft-cooked egg
    1 slice salt-free toast
    1 tsp salt-free margarine
    4 oz milk
    other drinks: see chapter introduction

LUNCH:

    2 oz salt-free baked fish
    1/2 cup salt-free egg noodles
    1/2 cup salt-free brown beans
    1/2 cup salt-free canned pear halves without juice
    1 slice salt-free bread
    1 tsp salt-free butter
    4 oz milk
    other drinks: see chapter introduction

DINNER:

    1 cup salt-free cottage cheese and pears
    1 slice salt-free bread
    1 tsp salt-free margarine
    1/2 cup canned pineapple without juice
    4 oz milk
    other drinks: see chapter introduction

SNACK:

    2 tsp shelled unsalted walnuts
    6 oz milk

DAYS 19 AND 49

BREAKFAST:

1/2 100-mg vitamin C tablet
4 oz grape juice
2 slices salt-free bread
1 tsp salt-free butter
4 oz milk
other drinks: see chapter introduction

LUNCH:

2 oz salt-free sliced beef
1 oz salt-free gravy
1/2 cup salt-free mashed potatoes
1/2 cup canned carrots
1 slice salt-free bread
1/2 cup raspberry ice cream (store bought, salt-free)
4 oz milk
other drinks: see chapter introduction

DINNER:

2 oz salt-free cornish hen*
1 oz cranberry sauce
1 oz salt-free gravy
1/2 cup sweet potatoes and apples
1/2 cup salt-free green beans
1 slice salt-free bread
1 tsp salt-free margarine
1/2 cup applesauce
drinks: see chapter introduction

SNACK:

6 oz milk
2 pieces rusk
1 3-oz piece salt-free cheese

DAYS 20 AND 50

BREAKFAST:

    1/2 100-mg vitamin C tablet
    4 oz apple juice
    1 salt-free soft-cooked egg
    1 slice salt-free toast
    1 tsp salt-free margarine
    4 oz milk
    other drinks: see chapter introduction

LUNCH:

    2 oz salt-free boiled mollusk (shelled fish, such as clams, squid, etc. Throw away whiter part.)
    1/2 cup salt-free white rice
    1/2 cup salt-free asparagus
    1 slice salt-free bread
    1 tsp salt-free butter
    1 slice salt-free homemade apple pie*
    4 oz milk
    other drinks: see chapter introduction

DINNER:

    4 oz salt-free spaghetti and meat balls
    1/2 cup salt-free green beans
    1/2 cup salt-free custard* (no chocolate)
    4 oz milk
    other drinks: see chapter introduction

SNACK:

    6 oz milk
    1 salt-free homemade pastry

DAYS 21 AND 51

BREAKFAST:

1/2 100-mg vitamin C tablet
4 oz apple juice
1 slice salt-free toast
1 tsp salt-free butter
4 oz milk
other drinks: see chapter introduction, add 1 tsp sugar if desired

LUNCH:

2 oz salt-free roast chicken
1 oz salt-free gravy
1/2 cup salt-free white rice
1/2 cup carrots
1 tsp salt-free butter
1/2 cup salt-free strawberry ice cream
4 oz milk
other drinks: see chapter introduction

DINNER:

2 oz salt-free roast beef
1 oz salt-free gravy
1 salt-free small baked potato
1/2 cup salt-free peas
1 slice salt-free bread
1 tsp salt-free butter
1/2 cup applesauce
4 oz milk
other drinks: see chapter introduction

SNACK:

2 slices pineapple
6 oz milk

DAYS 22 AND 52

BREAKFAST:

1/2 100-mg vitamin C tablet
4 oz apple juice
1 salt-free soft-cooked egg
1 slice salt-free toast
1 tsp salt-free jam or jelly
4 oz milk
other drinks: see chapter introduction

LUNCH:

2 oz salt-free steak
1 oz salt-free gravy
1/2 cup salt-free noodles
1/2 cup salt-free drained green beans
1 slice salt-free bread
1 tsp salt-free butter
1/2 cup canned pineapple without juice
4 oz milk
other drinks: see chapter introduction

DINNER:

2 oz salt-free baked fish fillet
1 salt-free small boiled potato
1/2 cup salt-free asparagus
1 slice salt-free bread
1 tsp salt-free butter
1/2 cup custard* (except chocolate)
4 oz milk
other drinks: see chapter introduction

SNACK:

1 salt-free homemade pineapple pastry
6 oz milk

DAYS 23 AND 53

BREAKFAST:

1/2 100-mg vitamin C tablet
4 oz apple juice
1 salt-free soft-cooked egg
1 slice salt-free toast
1 tsp salt-free butter
4 oz milk
other drinks: see chapter introduction

LUNCH:

2 oz salt-free chopped beef
1/2 cup salt-free white rice
1/2 cup salt-free green beans
lettuce, salt-free salad dressing
1 slice salt-free bread
1 tsp salt-free butter
1/2 cup lime gelatin dessert
4 oz milk
other drinks: see chapter introduction

DINNER:

2 oz salt-free sirloin
1 oz salt-free gravy
1/2 cup salt-free noodles
1/2 cup salt-free canned carrots
1 slice salt-free bread
1 tsp salt-free butter
1/2 cup drained canned pears
4 oz milk
other drinks: see chapter introduction

SNACK:

1 slice salt-free homemade apple pie*
6 oz milk

DAYS 24 AND 54

BREAKFAST:

1/2 100-mg vitamin C tablet
4 oz grape juice
1 salt-free soft-cooked egg
1 slice salt-free toast
1 tsp salt-free butter or jelly
4 oz milk
other drinks: see chapter introduction

LUNCH:

2 oz salt-free roast lamb
1 oz salt-free gravy
1/2 cup salt-free rice
1/2 cup salt-free summer squash
1 slice salt-free bread
1 tsp salt-free butter
4 oz milk
other drinks: see chapter introduction

DINNER:

2 oz salt-free turkey
1 oz salt-free gravy
1/4 cup salt-free mashed potato
1/2 cup salt-free corn
1 slice salt-free bread
1 tsp salt-free butter
1/2 cup canned pears (without juice)
4 oz milk
other drinks: see chapter introduction

SNACK:

1 salt-free homemade pastry
6 oz milk

DAYS 25 AND 55

BREAKFAST:

1/2 100-mg vitamin C tablet
4 oz apple juice
1 salt-free soft-boiled egg
1 slice salt-free toast
1 tsp salt-free butter or jam
4 oz milk
other drinks: see chapter introduction

LUNCH:

2 oz salt-free chicken
1 oz salt-free gravy
1/2 cup salt-free white rice
1/2 cup salt-free green beans
1 slice salt-free bread
1 tsp salt-free butter
1/2 cup canned halved peaches without juice
4 oz milk
other drinks: see chapter introduction

DINNER:

2 oz salt-free rolled flounder*
1 oz salt-free egg sauce*
1/2 cup salt-free duchess potatoes*
1/2 cup salt-free peas
1 slice salt-free bread
1 tsp salt-free butter
1/2 cup applesauce
4 oz milk
other drinks: see chapter introduction

SNACK:

1/2 cup custard* (except chocolate)
6 oz milk

DAYS 26 AND 56

BREAKFAST:

1/2 100-mg vitamin C tablet
4 oz grape juice
1 salt-free omelet
1 slice salt-free toast
1 tsp salt-free jam or jelly
4 oz milk
other drinks: see chapter introduction

LUNCH:

2 oz salt-free sliced beef
2 tbsp salt-free gravy from the beef
1/2 cup salt-free spaghetti
1/2 cup salt-free asparagus
1 slice salt-free bread
1 tsp salt-free butter
1/2 cup yogurt
4 oz milk
other drinks: see chapter introduction

DINNER:

2 oz salt-free beef
1 salt-free baked potato
1/2 cup salt-free green beans
1 slice salt-free bread
1 tsp salt-free butter
1/2 cup salt-free cottage cheese
4 oz milk
other drinks: see chapter introduction

SNACK:

1 3-oz piece salt-free cheese
1 salt-free cracker

DAYS 27 AND 57

BREAKFAST:

1/2 100-mg vitamin C tablet
4 oz apple juice
1 salt-free poached egg
1 slice salt-free toast
1 tsp salt-free jam or jelly
4 oz milk
other drinks: see chapter introduction

LUNCH:

2 oz salt-free turkey
1 oz salt-free gravy
1/2 cup salt-free white rice
1/2 cup carrots
lettuce, salt-free salad dressing
1 slice salt-free bread
1 tsp salt-free butter
1/2 cup salt-free strawberry ice cream
4 oz milk
other drinks: see chapter introduction

DINNER:

2 oz salt-free veal
1 oz salt-free gravy
1/2 cup salt-free noodles
1/2 cup salt-free green beans
1/2 cup lettuce, salt-free salad dressing
1 slice salt-free bread
1 tsp salt-free butter
1/2 cup canned pineapple (without juice)
4 oz milk
other drinks: see chapter introduction

SNACK:

1 salt-free homemade pastry
6 oz milk

DAYS 28 AND 58

BREAKFAST:

1/2 100-mg vitamin C tablet
4 oz grape juice
1 salt-free soft-cooked egg
1 slice salt-free toast
1 tsp honey or jam
4 oz milk
other drinks: see chapter introduction

LUNCH:

2 oz salt-free baked fish
1/2 cup salt-free white rice
1/2 cup sliced carrots
1 slice salt-free bread
1 tsp salt-free butter
1/2 cup gelatin dessert
4 oz milk
other drinks: see chapter introduction

DINNER:

2 oz salt-free sliced lamb
1 salt-free small boiled potato
1/2 cup salt-free green beans
1 slice salt-free bread
1 tsp salt-free butter
1/2 cup yogurt
4 oz milk
other drinks: see chapter introduction

SNACK:

1 salt-free homemade pastry
6 oz milk

DAYS 29 AND 59

BREAKFAST:

    1/2 100-mg vitamin C tablet
    4 oz apple juice
    1 salt-free soft-cooked egg
    1 slice salt-free toast
    1 tsp salt-free butter
    4 oz milk
    other drinks: see chapter introduction

LUNCH:

    2 oz salt-free roast lamb
    1 salt-free mashed potato
    1/2 cup carrots
    1 slice salt-free bread
    1 tsp salt-free butter
    1/2 cup applesauce
    4 oz milk
    other drinks: see chapter introduction

DINNER:

    2 oz salt-free broiled steak
    1 oz salt-free gravy
    1/2 cup salt-free cucumbers
    1 slice salt-free bread
    1 tsp salt-free butter
    1/2 cup yogurt
    4 oz milk
    other drinks: see chapter introduction

SNACK:

    1/2 cup custard* (except chocolate)
    6 oz milk

DAYS 30 AND 60

BREAKFAST:

    1/2 100-mg vitamin C tablet
    4 oz grape juice
    1 salt-free soft-cooked egg
    1 slice salt-free toast
    1 tsp salt-free butter or margarine
    4 oz milk
    other drinks: see chapter introduction

LUNCH:

    2 oz salt-free broiled chicken
    1 oz salt-free gravy
    1 salt-free mashed potato
    1/2 cup salt-free pared raw cucumber
    1 slice salt-free bread
    1 tsp salt-free butter
    1 pear
    4 oz milk
    other drinks: see chapter introduction

DINNER:

    2 oz salt-free baked fish fillet
    1 small salt-free baked potato
    1/2 cup salt-free green beans
    1 slice salt-free bread
    1 tsp salt-free butter
    1/2 cup gelatin dessert
    4 oz milk
    other drinks: see chapter introduction

SNACK:

    1 slice salt-free homemade strawberry pie*
    6 oz milk

Recipes for Girls and Boys 8

YOU PROBABLY CAME across some dishes in either the boy or girl diet that you didn't recognize—or, at any rate, that you didn't know how to cook. We can't promise you a comprehensive cookbook here, but the following recipes should help you prepare some of the more complex of the dishes. If you have any questions about the ingredients or cooking procedures for any of the other items on the suggested menus, you can find the answers in any good, basic cookbook.

For your convenience, these recipes are divided into two broad categories: *(a)* main dishes and *(b)* other dishes, a heading that includes such items as desserts, appetizers, and vegetables.

MAIN DISHES

VEAL AND PEPPER: Use 2 medium green peppers, 3 tbs vegetable oil or butter, 1 or 2 medium-size onions, 2 cups peeled tomatoes, 1 tsp salt. Sauté the onions, peppers, and tomatoes in the butter. Add 8 oz of veal to it, and as you sauté, add 1 chicken bouillon cube and a little water. Simmer on low heat on top burner for 10–15 minutes.

PINK SALMON: Use 1 tsp butter or vegetable oil, 1 medium-size onion, 2 peeled tomatoes, 1 tsp salt. Cut onion, 1 green pepper, and tomatoes into pieces. Sauté green pepper, onions, and tomatoes. Add 2 oz of tomato paste. Add 8 oz of canned salmon. Simmer for 10 minutes.

CORNISH HEN: This is chicken cooked when young. Season the hen with pepper and salt, rub a little butter on the top of it, and bake in the oven for 50 minutes at 375 degrees F.

HAWAIIAN CHICKEN: Cut chicken into 2 parts, boil for about 20 minutes, then remove it and dip it in wheat flour. Finally, fry it briefly to a golden brown in deep corn oil to give it a special flavor. Garnish with heated canned pineapple cubes.

YANKEE POT ROAST: Season roast with salt, pepper, and a little garlic. Then rub it with butter and bake in oven for 20 to 30 minutes for each 8 oz of meat at 375 degrees F.

SARDINE SALAD WITH GARNISH: Use 3 oz canned sardines, some lettuce, and a green pepper. Arrange it to suit your aesthetic tastes.

SALMON SALAD COLD PLATE: Arrange lettuce, 4 oz canned salmon, and decorate with 4 olives.

ROLLED FISH: Use boneless fresh fish. Bake it in oven for 20 minutes at 375 degrees F. You can also use an egg sauce made with 1 egg, 1/4 cup milk, and 1 tsp flour. Mix egg, flour, and milk together. Boil for 10 minutes and pour on fish.

ASPARAGUS SOUFFLÉ: Use several stalks of asparagus and a green pepper. Separate the yolk and the white of an egg. Add *no* salt. You grind the asparagus and the pepper, beat the egg yolk, pour the egg yolk on top and mix with the ground asparagus and pepper. Then, fry it in a little butter. Finally, stir lightly and serve.

LIVER: Put salt-free margarine or butter on a strip of liver and set it aside. Sauté sliced onion and green pepper. Do *not* add salt. Then, add the liver strip, and fry it for 10–15 minutes longer.

SHORT RIBS: Boil ribs first in water; then spread a little butter on them and put into oven to brown.

POTTED SWISS STEAK: Use 4 oz steak meat, sliced 3/4 inch thick, then cut into small portions. Mix flour, salt, and pepper. Pound this mixture into meat. Brown meat in fat, then place on baking pan and bake in an oven at 250 degrees F for 40 minutes.

HONEY-DRIP CHICKEN: Use flour, salt, and poultry seasoning (from store). Cut chicken into pieces of desired size. Roll chicken pieces in seasoned flour. Brown chicken in hot fat about one-half inch deep in pan. Reduce heat and cook slowly until tender (usually 20–30 minutes). Turn the chicken as necessary to assure even browning and doneness, and as you turn, gradually drip 2–3 tbs of honey on the chicken.

CHICKEN FRICASSEE: Use a whole or part chicken, flour, salt, pepper, and fats. Cut chicken into desired pieces. Dip each piece in seasoned flour. Brown in hot fat. Remove from the frying pan and in another pan cover the chicken with boiling water. Cook slowly on the stove, adding more water if necessary. When tender, remove chicken from stock (the water from the chicken); make gravy by using liquid in which chicken was cooked. Serve gravy over the chicken.

A VARIATION ON THIS DISH: Sprinkle with sliced ripe olives and sautéed fresh mushrooms.

BEANS SUPREME: Use 1 cup of navy beans. Wash beans, add boiling water, cover, and let stand 1 hour or longer. Cook in some water until tender, usually about 1 hour. Add more water as necessary. Then, add all these ingredients to the beans: 1 oz salt, 2 oz brown sugar, 1/2 tsp mustard, 1 tbs vinegar, 1/2 cup molasses, 1/2 cup catsup (optional), 4 oz cube salt pork (optional, available in store). Pour beans into deep baking pan and bake for 3–4 hours at 350 degrees F.

BAKED LIMA BEANS: Ingredients are 2 oz lima beans, 2 cups water, 2 oz chopped pimiento, 2 oz bacon fat, 1/2 tsp salt, 1/2 cup molasses, and a salt pork slice. Wash beans, add boiling water, and cook beans on top of stove until tender. Then add seasoning, pour into baking pan, and place salt pork on top of the beans. Finally, bake until brown (this takes about 1 hour) at 350 degrees F.

OTHER DISHES

PUMPKIN: Dice it, then bake at 375 degrees F for 20–25 minutes or boil 15–20 minutes.

SPANISH RICE: Use one green pepper, 1/2 cup diced onions, one-half can tomato paste, 1/2 cup canned tomatoes, seasoning (chicken cube), and 1/2 cup rice. You cut up and mix the green pepper, onions, and tomatoes and sauté them in cooking oil or butter. Then add the tomato paste, chicken cube, and a cup of water. Finally, add the rice and then boil for 15–20 minutes on low heat.

FIESTA COLESLAW: It's a 1/2 cup mixture of green peppers and pimiento (red), sliced together.

FRIED MUSHROOMS: Season mushrooms with salt and pepper and fry in corn oil in pan.

DUCHESS POTATOES: Boil potatoes, mash them, add a little milk, and mix the potatoes up.

EGG SAUCE: Separate yolks from whites of 2 eggs. Set aside. Melt 1 tsp butter in saucepan; blend in 1 tbsp flour. Add 1 cup milk, 2 egg yolks and dash of pepper and cook over low heat for 10 minutes, stirring often.

CUSTARD: Use 1 egg, 2 tsp sugar, 1/2 cup cold milk. Beat egg slightly, add sugar and cold milk, mix with low-speed blender until blended, and pour into custard cup. Refrigerate immediately, or bake at 375 degrees F for 10 to 15 minutes. (Then chill it if you like.)

HOMEMADE PIE: For top and bottom crusts, use 4 oz flour, 6 oz margarine or butter (salt-free for girls), 1/4 cup cold water. Add water to flour and fat, and mix together. Apportion flour mixture into 2 bowls for top and bottom crust. Put in refrigerator for about 10 minutes before rolling. Line pie pan with pastry. Put ample filling (such as apples, strawberries, raspberries, or other fruit, with the juice strained away) into unbaked bottom crust. Moisten edge of bottom crust. Cover with perforated top crust. Seal edge; bake for 30 minutes at 400 degrees F.

Conclusion: Now It's Up to You!

WHEN WE STARTED this adventure together, one of the first points mentioned was how deeply this issue of selecting the sex of a baby can delve into basic parental emotions.

We often want a child of a certain gender, but we're not quite sure why—at least not until we've identified exactly what it is we're feeling and tried to understand why we feel that way. One of the best ways to deal with difficult emotions is to learn to communicate how we feel to friends and loved ones. So one of the underlying purposes of this book has been to try to foster increased communication between a prospective mother and father—at the same time that they increase their chances for a child of the desired sex.

In pursuing the diet approach to preconception gender selection, it's extremely important for both the man and the woman to discuss not only whether they want a boy or a girl but also *why* they want what they want. In this sensitive area, everybody's feelings are equally valid. There is no way that anyone can make an absolutely definitive, convincing argument for either a boy or a girl.

But there are many ways that prospective parents, through meaningful interaction and conversation, can improve their relationship and prepare themselves for parenthood and a rewarding family life. A diet of the type presented in this book, with which the man and woman decide what sex they want and then both commit themselves to the same healthy eating pattern, is tailor-made to enhance this sort of communication.

But our interest in you doesn't end with this final chapter. In fact, we'd like for *you* to write the final chapter by letting us know if you decide to go on this diet. It's important that we hear from you *before* you have your baby to make our further study in this area most helpful, so we'd appreciate it if you would send us the following information on a separate sheet of paper:

Your name _____

Your address _____

_____

Your telephone number ( ) _____

What sex do you want your baby to be? _____

Does the father of the child plan to follow the mother's diet? _____

Please send this information to us at the following address:

Proctor & Langendoen
P.O. Box 4025, Grand Central Station
New York, N.Y. 10163

Also, be sure to send us a birth announcement when your baby arrives!

But no matter which sex your baby is, we know the experience you'll have preparing for childbirth and bolstering your health before pregnancy with a balanced diet will make it far easier to be a good parent. After all, the important thing is ultimately not whether you have a boy or girl, but whether you have the capacity to show boundless love to the new little addition to your life.

APPENDIX
Food Exchanges for Boy and Girl Diets

EVERY DIET—whether for weight loss, cardiovascular problems, or, in the present case, preconception gender selection—presents problems for certain people. We realize, for example, that readers who live some distance from a major city or shopping area may have problems finding a few of the foods that have been listed in both the boy and the girl diets in the main part of this book. Others may find that a number of the suggested dishes simply don't suit their palates.

To remedy these problems, we have devised, in consultation with professional nutritionists, some lists of equivalent foods that can be substituted for those suggested in the boy and the girl diets. If you make these substitutions thoughtfully and *sparingly,* you'll still be able to keep within the general limits of the diets—and achieve the ultimate goal of increasing your chances of having a baby of the desired sex.

But it's important to keep the general content of each day's menu, as suggested in the text, intact. Remember: Great pains have been taken by nutritionists and other experts to be certain that these diets are well balanced, properly limited in calories, and weighted to favor certain minerals.

You'll notice that there are two separate sets of lists, one for the boy-diet substitutions and one for the girl-diet substitutions. We'll be saying more about making food exchanges, but as we do, always keep in mind: *All food substitutions must be made only within the context of one diet or the other.* If you exchange a "boy food," such as an avocado, for something on the girl diet, you'll undercut the main purpose of the diet, which is to influence the sex of your future baby.

In the following pages, foods similar in sodium, potassium, calcium, and magnesium content have been grouped together into the same food groups, known among nutritionists as "exchange lists." Foods within each group can be substituted in the amounts specified for other foods in that list.

As you'll see, each food exchange list contains many foods, including a broad selection of choices other than those listed on the suggested boy and girl menus. Also, the dishes are arranged so as to make the job of calculating changes in your diet easier. For example, you don't have to sit down and count milligrams of sodium, potassium, calcium, and magnesium from a nutritionist's food values book. It's only necessary that you choose a food item within a certain grouping (such as the vegetable grouping) and then substitute that particular food for one in the same grouping on one of the daily menus in the text.

Our nutritionists say that, generally speaking, any of these foods can be cooked in any style desired, unless there is a contrary indication in the listings. Now let's go directly to the food exchange lists and see how you can take an active role in tailoring your preconception diet to your special tastes.

FOOD EXCHANGES FOR THE BOY DIET

Before you even begin to think about substituting one food for another, it's important first to go back to chapter 6 and study the introduction to the standard menus carefully. There are many guidelines and cautionary notes contained in those pages that you should keep in mind as you're making exchanges. Here are the categories of "boy foods" with equivalent quantities of each food item in each category:

MEAT EXCHANGES:

    3 oz corned tongue
    3 oz pastrami
    3 oz ham—boiled, Virginia, or capocolla
    3 oz bacon burger
    3 oz pork
    3 medium sardines or anchovies
    3 oz pickled herring
    3 oz Canadian bacon
    3 oz gefilte fish
    3 oz salami, liverwurst, or Spam
    3 oz deviled ham
    6 tbls peanut butter
    3 oz pepperoni pizza
    3 oz halibut or flounder
    3 medium-size meatballs
    3/4 cup oil-packed tuna
    3 oz caviar
    3 hot dogs
    3 1/2 oz chili con carne
    6 meat ravioli
    3 oz lox
    3 oz chicken salad
    3 oz lean veal
    4 oz sauerbraten
    2 knockwurst

VEGETABLE EXCHANGES:

1 artichoke
1/2 cup celery (raw)
3/4 cup canned sauerkraut
1/2 cup Swiss chard
1/4 cup beets
1 7-inch carrot (raw)
1/2 cup frozen peas
1/4 avocado
1/2 cup frozen broccoli
1 corn on cob
1/4 cup dried beans—dry white, lentils, soy, lima
1 small potato
1 medium tomato
1/2 cup tomato or vegetable juice
1/2 cup mushrooms
1 pepper (green or red)
1/2 cup winter squash
1 cup cauliflower
3/4 cup rutabaga
1/2 cup asparagus, frozen in butter sauce or canned

FRUIT EXCHANGES:

1 banana
1/2 cantaloupe (or any melon)
2/3 cup fruit cocktail
1 cup grapefruit juice
1 cup orange juice
1 medium peach (fresh)—should measure about 1/2 cup
10 prunes
1 orange or 1 cup orange segments
2/3 cup prune juice
1 cup canned apricots
24 dates—should measure about 1 cup
1 cup grapefruit sections

1 cup orange and grapefruit juice combination
1 cup pineapple juice
2 raw plums
1 cup grape juice
3/4 cup raisins
10 strawberries—about 1/2 cup
3/4 cup rhubarb
4 kumquats
5 figs
2 large or 3 small chestnuts, roasted
1/4 medium papaya

SOUP EXCHANGES:

NOTE: In general, "cream" soups should be avoided, though it's acceptable to use those indicated below when they are canned and made with water rather than milk.

1/2 cup chicken matzo ball
1 cup vegetable
3/4 cup French onion, no cheese
3/4 cup canned cream of celery, made with water
1/2 cup canned cream of chicken, made with water
1/2 cup green pea
1/2 cup wonton
1/2 cup turkey noodle
1 cup canned cream of asparagus, made with water
1/2 cup bean with bacon
3/4 cup turkey vegetable
1 cup minestrone
1 cup tomato rice
Instant soups, one serving each (in envelopes):
Beef noodle
chicken noodle
green pea
onion
spring vegetable
tomato

BREAD AND STARCH EXCHANGES:

1 muffin, English or corn
1 small bagel
1 slice raisin bread
1 slice white bread
1 hamburger bun
1 frankfurter roll
1 cup croutons
2 breadsticks
1 tortilla
6 3-ring pretzels
6 saltines
12 Sociables
4 Uneeda biscuits
7 Ritz crackers
1/4 cup wheatgerm
1/4 cup baked beans (canned)
1 potato
1 biscuit
1/2 cup chow mein noodles
5 rectangles melba toast
15 potato chips
5 vanilla wafers
3 cups salted popcorn
1/2 cup french fries
1/2 cup sweet potato
1 slice banana bread
1/2 cup bread stuffing

Cereals, 3/4 cup each:

NOTE: The box labels on cereals must be carefully checked to ensure high potassium and salt and low calcium and magnesium for boy-baby diet.

Corn flakes
Bran flakes (e.g., Bran Flakes, All-Bran, Raisin Bran)
Special K
Rice Krispies

FAT EXCHANGES:

1 tsp butter
1 tsp margarine
1/8 avocado
5 small olives
2 tsp blue cheese dressing
2 tsp tartar sauce
2 tsp Thousand Island or Russian dressing
2 tsp sesame seeds
1 strip bacon
2 tbs light cream
1 tbs chitterlings
1 tbs Italian dressing
3/4-inch cube salt pork
2 tsp Sofrito
2 tsp mayonnaise
1 tbs cream cheese
1 tsp corn, sunflower, olive, peanut oils
2 tbs sunflower seeds

DESSERT EXCHANGES:

1 slice strawberry pie
1 slice cherry pie
1 slice pecan pie
2 oatmeal cookies
1 slice carrot cake
1 slice apple strudel
1/2 cup sherbet
1 blueberry turnover
1 piece lemon meringue pie
1 piece rhubarb pie
1 piece pumpkin pie
1 plain doughnut
2 raisin cookies
1 piece fruitcake
1 piece baklava

FOOD EXCHANGES FOR THE GIRL DIET

These food exchanges are based on the principles stated in the introduction to chapter 7. So if you want to have the best chance of conceiving a girl—and also of maintaining a well-balanced diet—be sure to study that section of the main text closely.

In particular, be certain that you remember to take one-half of a 100-milligram tablet of vitamin C each day so that you'll meet your minimum daily requirements for that vitamin. Also, remember that it's important to avoid foods or seasonings containing salt.

Here are the "girl baby" foods. As with the boy diet, the food items are listed in amounts that will enable you to substitute them *sparingly* for one another within each food category.

MEAT EXCHANGES:

2 oz chicken
2 oz Cornish hen
2 oz turkey
2 oz hamburger
2 1/2 oz lamb chops
2 1/2 oz duckling
2 oz haddock
1/2 cup salt-free cottage cheese
2 oz salt-free Swiss Lorraine cheese
2 oz boiled lobster meat (without juice)
1/2 cup water-packed tuna
2 oz filet mignon
2 oz veal chops
2 oz veal scallopini
2 oz boiled crab meat (without juice)
2 oz liver
2 oz fresh bass, halibut, flounder, trout
2 oz roast sirloin of beef
2 oz broiled steak
1/2 cup salt-free nuts
2 oz salt-free egg salad

VEGETABLE EXCHANGES:

1/2 cup wax beans
1/2 cup cooked fresh carrots, drained
10-16 sprigs watercress
1/2 cup cucumber
1/2 cup onion
2 scallions
3 radishes
1/2 cup summer squash
1/2 cup asparagus
1 cup eggplant
1/2 cup canned bamboo shoots
1/2 cup cooked Brussels sprouts, drained
3/4 cup fresh green beans, cooked in water
5-6 leaves lettuce
5-6 leaves escarole, endives, or chicory
1 cup cooked cauliflower, drained
1/2 cup peas
1 cup alfalfa sprouts

FRUIT EXCHANGES:

1 small apple
1/2 cup apple juice
3/4 cup applesauce
1/2 cup blackberries, fresh or frozen
1/2 cup blueberries, fresh or frozen
1 cup cranberries
1 pear, canned without juice
1 peach, canned without juice
1 cup pear nectar
1 tangerine
1 slice raw pineapple
12 grapes
1/3 cup canned pineapples, without juice
1/2 cup mandarin oranges (*not* Florida oranges)

BREAD AND STARCH EXCHANGES:

NOTE: All these foods must be prepared without salt.

1 slice Italian bread
1 slice rye bread
1 slice whole-wheat bread
2 graham crackers
1/2 cup cooked macaroni, noodles, or spaghetti
1 plain roll
5 low-sodium crackers
2 matzo, plain and unsalted
1/2 cup egg barley
1 slice pumpernickel
1 slice French bread
3 zwieback
12 Wheat Thins
3 cups unsalted popcorn
2 tbs cornmeal
1 cup rice
1/3 cup corn
1/2 cup shredded wheat
3/4 cup puffed wheat or puffed rice
1/2 cup buckwheat cereal
1 French toast with syrup
1 popover
1 slice hallah bread
1/2 cup salt-free bread stuffing

FAT EXCHANGES:

1 tsp salt-free butter
1 tsp salt-free margarine
10–15 salt-free peanuts
2 tbs sour cream
1 tbs heavy cream
2 tsp salt-free mayonnaise
2–3 tsp salt-free salad dressings (French, Italian)
2 tbs light cream

DAIRY EXCHANGES:

Nonfat fortified milk:
1 cup skim or nonfat milk
1/2 cup canned evaporated skim milk
1/3 cup powdered nonfat dry milk
1 cup buttermilk from skim milk
1 cup yogurt from skim milk (unflavored)

Lowfat fortified milk:
1 cup 2%-fat fortified milk
1 cup 1%-fat fortified milk
1 cup yogurt from 2%-fat fortified milk (unflavored)

Whole milk:
1 cup whole milk
1/2 cup canned evaporated whole milk
1 cup buttermilk from whole milk
1 cup yogurt from whole milk (unflavored)

Bibliography

Antia, F. P. *Clinical Dietetics and Nutrition.* 2nd ed. New York: Oxford University Press, 1973.
"Babymaking: Dress Them in Blue." *Science News,* 12 January 1974, pp. 20–21.
Beeson, Paul, et al., eds. *Cecil Textbook of Medicine.* 15th ed. Philadelphia: W. B. Saunders Company, 1979.
Blackman, Ann. "Want a Boy Baby? Or a Girl?" *Supplementary Material from The New York Times News Service and The Associated Press,* 6 September 1978, pp. 52ff.
"Boy or Girl, Take Your Pick." *Science Digest,* April 1974, pp. 17–18.
Brewer, Gail Sforza, and Brewer, Tom. *What Every Pregnant Woman Should Know: The Truth About Diets and Drugs in Pregnancy.* New York: Random House, 1977.
Brody, Jane E. "Feeding the Unborn: Some Diet Wisdom for Mothers-to-Be." *The New York Times,* 28 November 1979, Section III, p. 1.
Campbell, Colin. "What Happens When We Get the Manchild Pill?" *Psychology Today,* August 1976, p. 86.

"Choose the Sex of Your Baby? Maybe." *Good Housekeeping*, February 1979, p. 246.
"Choosing the Baby's Sex." *British Medical Journal* 280 (1980): 272–273.
Figes, Eva. "The Man-Child Fixation." *Ms.*, February 1974, pp. 74–75.
Gage, Joan. "It's Not Nice to be Fooled by Mother Nature." *The New York Times*, 31 August 1977, Section III, p. 14.
Galton, Lawrence. "Decisions, Decisions, Decisions." *The New York Times Magazine*, 20 June 1974, pp. 22ff.
"The Genetic Basis of Sex Determination." *Science News*, 6 December 1975, p. 356.
Glass, Robert H. "Sex Preselection." *Obstetrics and Gynecology* 49 (1977): 122–126.
Gordon, A. D. G. "Bicarbonate for a Boy, Vinegar for a Girl." *Nursing Times*, 74 (1978): 764–765.
Harriman, Sarah. *The Book of Ginseng*. New York: A Jove Book, 1973.
Horn, Jack. "The Secret of Sex Determination: Take It Easy." *Psychology Today*, November 1974, p. 139.
The Implications of Sex Preselection." *Technology Review*, March–April 1980, pp. 76–77.
Isselbacher, Kurt, et al., eds. *Harrison's Principles of Internal Medicine*. 9th ed. New York: McGraw-Hill Book Company, 1980.
Jaffin, Herbert. "Nutrition in Pregnancy." In *Quick Reference to Clinical Nutrition*, edited by Seymour L. Halpern. Philadelphia: J. B. Lippincott Company, 1979.
Lake, Alice. "Selecting the Sex of Babies: The New Moral Dilemma." *McCall's*, July 1976, pp. 47–48.
Lindeman, Robert D. "Minerals in Medical Practice." In *Quick Reference to Clinical Nutrition*, edited by Seymour L. Halpern. Philadelphia: J. B. Lippincott Company, 1979.
Lorrain, Jacques. "Pre-conceptional Sex Selection." *International Journal of Gynaecology and Obstetrics* 13 (1975): 127–130.
Massachusetts General Hospital Dietary Department. *Diet Manual*. Boston: Little, Brown, and Company, 1976.
Mayo Clinic Diet Manual. 3rd ed. Philadelphia: W. B. Saunders Company, 1961.

Muehleis, M. S., and Long, Sally Y. "The Effects of Altering the pH of Seminal Fluid on the Sex Ratio of Rabbit Offspring." *Fertility and Sterility* 27 (1976): 1438–1445.

"Nutritional Time Bomb." *Chemistry* 48 (1975): 27.

Rinzler, Carol Ann. *The Dictionary of Medical Folklore*. New York: Ballantine Books, 1979.

Robinson, Corinne H. *Normal and Therapeutic Nutrition*. 14th ed. New York: Macmillan, 1972.

Rorvik, David M. (with Shettles, Landrum B.). *Choose Your Baby's Sex*. New York: Dodd, Mead, 1977.

———. (with Shettles, Landrum B.). *Your Baby's Sex: Now You Can Choose*. New York: Dodd, Mead, 1970.

Rose, Kathryn. "Can You Pre-Select the Sex of Your Child?" *Harper's Bazaar*, July 1975, pp. 6–7.

Rosenzweig, Saul, and Adelman, Stuart. "Parental Predetermination of the Sex of Offspring: The Attitudes of Young Married Couples With University Education." *Journal of Biosocial Science* 8 (1976): 335–346.

Rosner, Fred. "The Biblical and Talmudic Secret for Choosing One's Baby's Sex." *Israel Journal of Medical Sciences* 15 (1979): 784–787.

"Selecting the Sex of Your Infant." *Science News*, 3 March 1979, p. 135.

"Sex Selection Before Child's Conception." *Journal of the American Medical Association* 241 (1979): 1220.

"Sex Selection: Technique Not Confirmed." *Science News*, 8 March 1975, p. 151.

Stolkowski, Joseph, and Lorrain, Jacques. "Preconceptional Selection of Fetal Sex." *International Journal of Gynaecology and Obstetrics* 18 (1980): 440–443.

United Nations. "Natality Statistics, 27th Issue." In *Demographic Yearbook*. New York: UN Publicity Service, 1975.

Vanderbilt University Dietary Staff. *Diet Manual*. 2nd ed. Nashville: Vanderbilt University Press, 1969.

Vear, Cedric S. "Preselective Sex Determination." *Medical Journal of Australia* 2 (1977): 700–702.

Waring, Philippa. *A Dictionary of Omens and Superstitions*. New York: Ballantine Books, 1978.

Westoff, Charles F., and Rindfuss, Ronald R. "Sex Preselection in the United States: Some Implications." *Science*, 10 May 1974, pp. 633–636.

Whelan, Elizabeth M. *A Baby? . . . Maybe: A Guide to Making the Most Fateful Decision of Your Life*. rev. ed. New York: Bobbs-Merrill, 1980.

———. *Boy or Girl?* New York: Bobbs-Merrill, 1977.

———. "Sex Selection." *Harper's Bazaar*, November 1976, p. 102.

Williams, Sue Rodwell. *Nutrition and Diet Therapy*. 3rd ed. St. Louis: C. V. Mosby, 1977.

Williamson, Nancy E., et al. "Evaluation of an Unsuccessful Sex Preselection Clinic in Singapore." *Journal of Biosocial Science* 10 (1978): 375–388.

"X vs. Y." *Saturday Review World*, 9 March 1979, p. 8.

The Authors

SALLY LANGENDOEN became a registered nurse through the diploma nursing program at Massachusetts General Hospital and then earned her B.S. in nursing from Simmons College. She has also done two years of graduate work in the psychology and sociology of medicine at Ohio State University.

For the last ten years, Langendoen has been pursuing an independent practice in New York City as a childbirth educator and has instructed hundreds of couples in the Lamaze technique and other subjects relating to pregnancy. She has been featured for her work in publications like the *New York Daily News* and *Parade*. A teacher accredited by the American Society for Psychoprophylaxis in Obstetrics, Langendoen has also had an opportunity to practice personally what she preaches—as the mother of a thirteen-year-old son.

In addition to her work as a childbirth educator, Sally Langendoen is an experienced medical writer. A member of the

American Medical Writers Association, she has been editor for three years of an international monthly publication for professional nurses. She has also contributed numerous articles to professional journals and such popular magazines as *American Baby.*

WILLIAM PROCTOR, a graduate of Harvard College and Law School, is the author or coauthor of more than a dozen books on a wide range of topics, including psychology, religion, and finance. His works include *P.D.A.—Personal Death Awareness* (Prentice-Hall, 1976) with Dr. J. William Worden of Harvard Medical School. He also is presently collaborating with pollster George Gallup Jr. on a book focusing on the scientific approach to unusual near-death experiences.

Index

Abortion, 26–27
Adelman, Stuart, 17
Alcohol, 65
Amnioscentesis, 23, 24–25
Aristotle, 20
Artificial insemination, 38–40
Asparagus Soufflé, 133

Babylonian Talmud, 22
Baked Lima Beans, 135
Baking soda, 20, 31–32
Beans Supreme, 134
Bernard, Claude, 8
Bicarbonate of soda, 20, 31–32
Binden, 7
Bonellia, 42

Bread exchanges
 boy diet, 146
 girl diet, 150
Brewer, Gail, 59
Brewer, Tom, 59

Caffeine, 65
Calcium, 42–46, 51, 53–58, 60–62, 63, 65, 100
Capacitation, 7
Cattle, 43
Cervical mucus, 6
Chicken, 133, 134
Chicken Fricassee, 134
Chinese cooking, 51, 52
Coital positions, 20, 33, 35

160 INDEX

Coleslaw, 135
Cornish Hen, 133
Corona radiata, 7
Cowpeas, 20, 56–57
Crime rate, 29
Cumulus, 7
Custard, 56, 135
Czechoslovakia, 19

Dairy exchanges
  girl diet, 151
Demasio, Dorcas, 52, 64, 65, 99, 100
Dessert exchanges
  boy diet, 147
Desserts, 55–56, 100, 136
Dmowski, W. Paul, 39
Douche method, 31–32, 35, 37
Drano test, 23–24
Duchess Potatoes, 135

Egg Sauce, 135
England, 20, 49, 50
English common law, 16
Ericsson, Ronald J., 39

Fallopian tubes, 6
Fat exchanges
  boy diet, 147
  girl diet, 150
Female firstborn, 17
Fertilization, 6–8, 31, 47
Fetal sex identification, 27
Fiesta Coleslaw, 135
Figes, Eva, 28
Firstborn, 16–17, 29

Fish, 18, 55, 133
Folklore, 18–24, 54–57
Fried Mushrooms, 135
Fruit exchanges
  boy diet, 144–145
  girl diet, 149

Gage, Joan, 24
Ghana, 18, 54
Ginseng root, 19
Glass, Robert, 38
Gordon, A. D. G., 32
Greece, 49, 51, 52
Greeks, ancient, 18, 20
Guerrero, Rodrigo, 35–38

Hebrew tradition, 21–22, 33
Heirs, 16
Henry VIII, 16
Herbst, Curt, 42
Hippocrates, 18
Homemade Pie, 136
Homosexuality, 28
Honey-Drip Chicken, 134
Hong Kong, 50, 52
Hungary, 19
Hypercalcemia, 61
Hypertension, 45, 59
Hypocalcemia, 61
Hypokalemia, 60

Intercourse, 33
  timing of, 33–38
Ions, 43–44, 46–47
Iron, 54, 55
Israel, 50, 52

INDEX

Japan, 49, 50
Jews, 21–22, 33, 49, 50, 51–52

Korea, 49
Kosher cooking, 51–52

Landers, Ann, 24
Lean, T. H., 36–37
Lettuce, 19
Lima beans, 135
Lion's blood, 20, 56
Liver, 134
Lorrain, Jacques, 43–48, 59–63

Magnesium, 42–46, 53, 58, 62, 63, 65, 100
Main dishes, 132–135
Male firstborn, 16–17
Mandrake root, 18–19
Marine worm, 42
Meat, 55
Meat exchanges
 boy diet, 143
 girl diet, 148
Mushrooms, 135

Navy beans, 134

Orgasm, 22–23, 33, 35
Ovulation, 34, 37, 40
Oysters, 18, 51, 54, 55

Parmenides, 20
pH (vagina), 32
Pies, 56, 136
Pink Salmon, 133
Positions, coital, 20, 33, 35
Pot roast, 133
Potassium, 42–47, 51, 53–58, 60, 65, 67, 100
Potatoes, 135
Potted Swiss Steak, 134
Proteolytic enzymes, 7
Pumpkin, 135

Rape, 21
Ratio, male-female, 48–53
 imbalance, 28–29
Receptors, 46–47
Restaurant menus, 66–67
Rice, 135
Rindfuss, Ronald, 28
Rolled Fish, 133
Rome, 19
Rorvik, David, 33, 36
Rosenzweig, Saul, 17
Rosner, Fred, 22
Russell, W. T., 49

Salmon, Pink, 133
Salmon Salad Cold Plate, 133
Salt. *See* Sodium
Sardine Salad with Garnish, 133
Schenk, Leopold, 41
Schuster, Donald, 21
Schuster, Locky, 21
Sex-linked disorders, 17
Shettles, Landrum, 5, 32–38
Short Ribs, 134

INDEX

Sodium, 43–47, 51, 53, 54, 55–56, 58–60, 65, 67, 99, 100
Soup exchanges
  boy diet, 145
Spanish Rice, 135
Sperm, 5–8, 30–31, 32, 34, 39, 45–46, 47
Starch exchanges
  boy diet, 146
  girl diet, 150
Stolkowski, Joseph, 43–48, 59–63
Superstitions, 18–24
Sweets, 55–56, 100, 136
Swiss steak, 134

Talmudic method, 21–22, 33
Twins, 19

Ulam, 22
Unterberger, Felix, 31

Veal and Pepper, 132–133
Vear, Cedric S., 35

Vegetable exchanges
  boy diet, 144
  girl diet, 149
Vengadasalam, D., 36–37

Wars, threat of, 29
Weather, 20
Welsh superstition, 23
Westoff, Charles, 28
Whelan, Elizabeth, 32, 35–36
Williamson, Nancy, 36–37
Wine, 20, 56

X sperm, 5, 30–31, 32, 39, 46, 47

Y sperm, 5, 30–31, 32, 34, 39, 45–46, 47
Yankee Pot Roast, 133

Zona pellucida, 7

CANCELLED